European Medicines
Pricing and Reimbursement

Now and the future

European Medicines Pricing and Reimbursement

Now and the future

Edited by

MARTINA GARAU
Economist, Office of Health Economics

and

JORGE MESTRE-FERRANDIZ
Senior Economist, Office of Health Economics

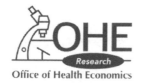

Office of Health Economics

Radcliffe Publishing
Oxford • Seattle

Radcliffe Publishing Ltd
18 Marcham Road
Abingdon
Oxon OX14 1AA
United Kingdom

www.radcliffe-oxford.com
Electronic catalogue and worldwide online ordering facility.

British Library Cataloguing in Publication Data
A catalogue record for this book is available from the British Library.

ISBN-10: 1 84619 184 X
ISBN-13: 978 1 84619 184 8

Typeset by Egan Reid Ltd, Auckland, New Zealand
Printed and bound by TJI Digital, Padstow, Cornwall

Contents

List of figures

List of tables

List of contributors

Dr Joan Costa-i-Font
University of Barcelona, Spain, and London School of Economics, UK

Professor Patricia Danzon
University of Pennsylvania, US

Dr Livio Garattini
CESAV, Centre for Health Economics of the Mario Negri Institute, Italy

Martina Garau
Office of Health Economics, UK

Professor Claude Le Pen
University of Paris-Dauphine and Aremis Consultants, France

Professor J-Matthias Graf von der Schulenburg
University of Hanover, Germany

Professor Adrian Towse
Office of Health Economics, UK

Introduction

Improving the regulatory framework for European pharmaceutical markets is a complex task which requires the achievement of several, sometimes competing objectives and involves the interests of a range of different stakeholders. The majority of European Union (EU) countries facing rising expenditure for healthcare endeavours to contain costs by controlling the price and/or volume of pharmaceuticals. Simultaneously, they also have to allow for patients' and clinicians' demands for access to high quality treatments, and for the promotion of an innovative and successful pharmaceutical industry.

Different approaches to balance these objectives of health and industrial policy have been implemented by member states, reflecting different national policy priorities and the particular features of national healthcare systems (e.g. level of health expenditures, healthcare financing system).

The chapters of this book are based on presentations given at a conference in London in late 2005 organised by the Office of Health Economics. The aim is not only to understand and discuss the mix of regulatory measures introduced by national policy makers in order to achieve their goals, but also to ascertain how these policies have actually shaped and influenced the characteristics and functioning of national pharmaceutical markets. In particular, each author has provided an analysis of existing pricing and reimbursement arrangements operating in their own country and an outline of policy scenarios that might emerge in the next decade.

The following paragraphs provide a summary of the main targets of pricing and reimbursement (P&R) regulation in the five big EU pharmaceutical markets: France, Germany, Italy, Spain and the UK, based on the information provided in the subsequent chapters. The final chapter by Professor Patricia Danzon provides evidence of the impact of these policies on a number of variables, including price levels, and offers some recommendations on improving policies aimed at regulating prices of on-patent and generic medicines.

By distinguishing between *demand-side* and *supply-side* regulation, we are able to highlight the impacts different policies might have on pharmaceutical expenditure. Whilst supply-side policies have a direct or indirect effect on pharmaceutical prices, the demand-side policies influence volume prescribed.

Taking into account this taxonomy, several key common themes emerge across the five countries analysed in this book.

Some common themes

On the supply side, numerous regulatory measures have been introduced with the purpose of reducing or containing medicines' prices. These include the following.

▶ Price–volume agreements and other agreements between national health bodies and individual companies. For example, in France the Health Products Economic Committee is responsible for negotiating the price with companies once positive advice for reimbursement has been given. Criteria used for this negotiation include not only the clinical evaluation of each product but also sales volume, international prices, macroeconomic objectives and parallel exports threat. A product-by-product approach has also been adopted in Italy and Spain. For instance, in Italy, prices of all new drugs that receive market approval by the European Medicines Agency (EMEA) are set by an agreement between the national authority and the company concerned.

▶ Price cuts and other compulsory price freezes introduced by national regulators. The latest (2005) Pharmaceutical Price Regulation Scheme (PPRS) agreement in the UK imposed an across-the-board price cut of 7% on branded pharmaceuticals sold to the UK National Health Service (NHS). This approach has also been adopted by the other countries considered, in particular, Germany, which enforced a price freeze for two years running, and Spain, which introduced a 4.2% price reduction in 2005 for all products on the Spanish market that had been in the market for more than one year and not subject to the generic reference price system.

▶ International reference pricing, using an average of prices in a set of countries, usually selected on the basis of the price level sought by the payers. This mechanism has been formally adopted in a number of countries, and is used informally during pricing negotiations in others.

Alongside these supply-side measures, we also find the following policies affecting indirectly price levels.

‣ Reference pricing within the national markets determining the maximum reimbursement limit for pharmaceuticals assigned to the same group. All countries considered in this book except the UK have a reference price system in order to contain prices of medicines to healthcare payers. Methods used to calculate the reference price and the levels of equivalence applied to classify products vary between countries. The latter factor determines coverage and gives rise to levels 1, 2 and 3 of reference pricing, which are based on chemical, pharmacological and therapeutic equivalence, respectively. While Spain applies level 1 reference pricing (products with the same active ingredient), Germany has recently allowed for on-patent and off-patent drugs to be grouped together. The main drawbacks of this system are that it provides little incentive for companies to invest in R&D and can be complicated to apply at the individual level. For instance, a product included in a particular group might not be equivalent to other products of the same cluster for a particular patient because of different contraindications.

‣ Rate of return regulation, primarily used in the UK. The latest (2005) PPRS agreement has established a target for the companies' return on capital employed of 21% and allows for research and development (R&D), sales promotion and information costs. However, it is not a cost-plus system. The PPRS represents a policy mechanism introduced to attain both cost-containment and industrial policy objectives, attempting to ensure reasonable prices of medicines for the NHS but also to reward R&D.

In addition to these policy instruments, the five countries under examination have introduced complementary reimbursement regimes which also can have an effect on utilisation. These include the following.

‣ Positive and negative lists. Although all countries considered have introduced national formularies which list products that should be considered (i.e. positive list) or should not be considered (i.e. negative list) for reimbursement, the implementation and the importance of these regimens vary from country to country.

‣ The use of economic evaluations to help determine prices, reimbursement or simply to offer prescribing recommendations. Economic evaluations are expected to gain an increasing importance as a tool for conditional reimbursement processes. In the UK, health bodies have been established with the purpose of appraising systematically the cost-effectiveness of selected health technologies and make recommendations on their use within the NHS. In other major EU markets, reimbursed status is granted mainly on the basis of evidence on clinical efficacy and effectiveness but it seems very likely that considerations of the value-for-money offered by new treatments will play an increasingly important role in the future.

On the demand-side, a range of policy options has been advocated and implemented by countries in order to control health products' volumes. They target prescribers, dispensers and patients as follows.

▶ In terms of affecting prescribing behaviour, tools include financial and non-financial incentives aimed at encouraging a more efficient use of healthcare resources and influencing clinical practice. The UK has put in place a comprehensive regulatory system for doctors, which embeds the allocation of prescribing budgets to physicians, prescribing incentive schemes, and the provision of information and education campaigns and clinical practice guidelines. Spain and Italy have also attempted to introduce some type of prescribing budgets and prescribers' incentives but further initiatives may take place at the regional level.

▶ Related to dispensing behaviour, only a few European countries have introduced incentives for pharmacists to dispense generic products, whilst others, despite the efforts put in to expanding the generics market, still have a system where pharmacists are not given an incentive to dispense them. In the UK pharmacists buy generic products at a discounted price offered by manufacturers and are reimbursed at a fixed tariff price. Hence, generic companies compete on the price they sell to pharmacists to offer them larger profit margins and obtain higher market share. Savings generated by the competition among generic companies are captured by the NHS. In Italy and Spain, these savings usually do not arise.

▶ Regarding patient purchase choice, cost-sharing policies can take the form of patients' payment of a fixed fee per prescription or a proportion of the retail price of products with the purpose of encouraging a more efficient pattern of consumption and, more generally, of developing a culture of responsibility and awareness of costs among prescribers and final users. In France, for instance, a patient co-payment system has been adopted based on the classification awarded to the product.

Future trends in national P&R policies

The chapters in this book show the divergences existing among national healthcare systems, in particular among the principles underlying regulatory systems and the objectives they are meant to achieve. One example is the differences between the French and the UK systems. In France a two-tier approach is adopted, where reimbursement decisions are made on the basis of the observed clinical effectiveness and, subsequent to the reimbursement status being granted, the price is negotiated between the health authority and the company. On the other hand, in the UK there is no price regulation at launch but subsequently health bodies such as the National Institute for Health and Clinical Excellence (NICE) make decisions on the use of health products within the NHS taking account of both clinical and cost-effectiveness.

However, at least one common element is invoked in all countries: the implementation of a standardised and comprehensive method to measure innovation and identify valuable differences among products that payers may be willing to reward. Economic evaluation, and in particular health technology assessment (HTA), attempts to evaluate the relative value for money of health technologies and shows the trade-off between the cost of treatments and the corresponding health benefits. HTA may not be perfect but it will help evaluate the additional value brought by new products in relation to competitors, especially now that new drugs such as the biologics have been introduced into the market and have to be compared with existing compounds.

An increasing number of initiatives have been undertaken at the European level with the purpose of co-ordinating national practices and developing common HTA procedures. One such example is the European Network of Health Economic Evaluation Databases (EURO NHEED). However, there is still no consistency in the use of HTA for decision-making across European countries, concerning both the institutional requirements for economic evaluation and their impact on P&R decisions.

Overall, it seems very likely that the role played by HTA in national P&R arrangements will rise, although the way through which it will be incorporated into current regulatory frameworks will vary from country to country. In France economic evaluations are not currently taken into account explicitly but they are increasingly likely to be used by companies for price negotiations to show the additional value of their products. In Germany, if the coverage of the reference price system is extended as expected, then HTA will be used to provide recommendations on reference prices of medicine groups. In Italy, the dossier that companies submit to the health authorities includes an economic evaluation, which is expected to have an increasing influence on price and reimbursement decisions. In Spain, it is likely that P&R processes will incorporate economic evaluations, maybe through the agencies that have already been established at the regional level, such as those in Andalusia and Catalonia. In the UK, where cost–effectiveness analysis is explicitly used by health bodies to determine utilisation patterns within the NHS, attention will probably be focused on improvement of existing processes, that is, reducing the time required to reach decisions and improving guideline implementation.

Martina Garau
Office of Health Economics
UK

Jorge Mestre-Ferrandiz
Office of Health Economics
UK

CHAPTER 1

Pricing and reimbursement policies in France: current and future trends

Claude Le Pen

This chapter discusses the current situation in the French pharmaceutical market and offers some ideas about what to expect in the future.

Overview of the French pharmaceutical market

Pharmaceutical expenditure in France currently amounts to about €19 billion at ex-factory prices, representing €25–26 billion at retail prices. It is the fourth largest market, and has the highest per capita consumption, in the world. Each French person consumes on average around one unit, that is, pack of medicines per week.

The growth rate of pharmaceutical expenditure in France is moderate, at around 5% and 1% per annum in value and volume terms respectively (October 2004–October 2005). However, growth patterns are different for the on-patent reimbursed drugs segment, the out-of-patent market and the over-the-counter (OTC) market. Sales of reimbursed medicines still on patent are declining in terms of units

1

(−3% over the year) whilst remaining relatively flat in value terms (−0.4%). On the other hand, the growth rates for the out-of-patent reimbursed drugs, in terms of value and units, amount to 41% and 55%, respectively. This is mainly attributed to the increasing number of out-of-patent molecules. In addition, the OTC market is strongly declining, with a negative growth rate of 4.7% in value terms and a negative growth rate of 6.5% in volume terms. Regarding market shares, on-patent medicines represent around 72% of the total pharmaceutical market, while off-patent and OTC medicines represent 21% and 7%, respectively.

Sales in the hospital market are €5.7 billion at ex-factory list prices. The exact prices of hospital medicines are not known as they are negotiated privately between companies and hospitals. Also, 46% of this €5.7 billion (i.e. €2.6 billion) is prescribed for hospital outpatients: hospital doctors prescribe medicines, including anti-cancer and anti-HIV medicines, for non-hospitalised patients, which are then paid for by health insurance funds. This segment can be considered as a third market; the other two markets being the more 'standard' hospital and pharmacy markets. This so-called 'third market' is growing. In addition, 40% of hospital sales (i.e. €2.3 billion) are funded separately, either by the so-called special 'innovation budgets' or directly by health funds, as 'pass-through' costs. They are not included in the French diagnosis-related groups (DRG) system, which finances public and private hospitals.

Current trends in national P&R regulation

There are two price regimens in France. First, there is a 'free-pricing' segment of the market, which includes the market for OTC and hospital drugs, which are included in the DRG costs and where hospitals negotiate directly with companies. Second, there is a 'regulated price' segment with the pharmacy-reimbursed drugs and hospital drugs which are not included in the DRG system.

The institutional framework for the P&R system in France involves a two-step process. The first step relates to reimbursement, and the institution involved is the Transparency Commission. The second step of the institutional framework involves setting the price of the medicine, once positive advice for reimbursement has been given. This price is set by the Health Products Economic Committee, which is located within the Ministry of Health. The Health Products Economic Committee is composed of civil servants from various ministries, including the Ministry of Health and the Ministry of Finance and Industrial Affairs. This system is represented in Figure 1.1.

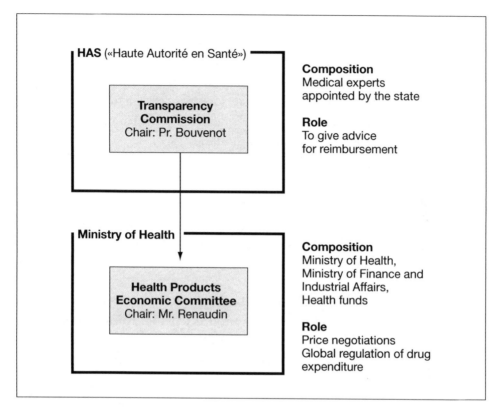

FIGURE 1.1   The institutional framework for the P&R system in France.

The Transparency Commission

The Transparency Commission has now been transferred from the Drug Agency to the new Agency for Quality of Care – *Haute Autorité en Santé* (HAS) – which has extended the Commission's responsibilities regarding the evaluation of drugs, medical devices, procedures and so on. The Transparency Commission is made up of medical experts appointed by the state and gives advice on reimbursement, with the Minister of Health being the last-resort decision-maker.

The Transparency Commission uses a very formal approach to drug evaluation. It gives advice based on the 'Rendered Medical Service' (SMR) and the 'Improvement in the Rendered Medical Service' (ASMR), representing two different criteria. The first criterion is static: what is the benefit of the drug? The second is dynamic: what improvement does the drug bring compared to existing treatment? For instance, a generic copy of a drug may render a high medical service without being an improvement.

Regarding the first criterion, the SMR, there is a link between the classification awarded to the product and the degree of co-payment borne by the patient. When a product receives the classification 'major' or 'important', the co-payment is set at 35% of the retail price; for medicines with an SMR deemed as 'moderate', the co-payment is higher (65%); and when a medicine is deemed to have a 'weak' or 'insufficient' SMR, the patient pays the full price, that is, the patient co-payment is 100%. The rating is based on the following criteria:

▶ efficacy/tolerance

▶ severity of the disease

▶ existence of therapeutic alternatives

▶ place in the therapeutic strategy (first-line, second-line, etc.)

▶ public health impact.

These items are defined by law, so for each medicine the Transparency Commission has to give advice on all of them. However, it is usually 'efficacy' and 'disease severity' that determine the medicine's classification. Indeed, usually 90% of the rating is determined by these two factors, while the other factors play a very minor role.

The 'ASMR' criterion is more dynamic, since it relates to a medicine's degree of innovation relative to the existing situation/available treatments. There are five possible grades to this classification: major (Level I); important (II); significant (III); minor (IV); no improvement (V). This rating is mainly based on direct comparative studies with the reference product, although indirect comparisons are sometimes allowed. The reference product is usually the most-sold medicine, the most recent and/or the most expensive in the new medicine's therapeutic class. The improvement is assessed on the basis of indication and population. For example, a medicine can generate an important improvement in some indications and patient groups but no improvement in others. In this case, the price is defined by the highest classification.

I will use verteporphin, which is a medicine for macular degeneration, as an example to illustrate how the system works. The advice was issued in 2003 for a new indication: age-related macular degeneration (ARMD) with 'occult subfoveal choroidal neovascularisation with evidence of recent or ongoing disease progression' (Eur. Reg. 22/8/2002). For this indication, the SMR was deemed by the Transparency Commission to be 'important', while the ASMR was classified as 'significant' – Level III.

The Transparency Commission also made a recommendation for the use of the product, a task that has been included in this body's remit only recently. This recommendation estimated the target population between 10 000 and 28 000 patients and set the date for a re-evaluation to be within 18 months, when new effectiveness evidence was expected to be available. The idea behind this re-evaluation is that the original evaluation is treated as a form of provisional authorisation based on clinical trials. The Transparency Commission needs real-life data in order to give a new authorisation.

The Transparency Commission examines about 500 dossiers each year, most of which concern new indications of already-marketed products (around 350 of the 500), while the rest deal with new products. Typically this classification system based on the level of innovation, as measured by the ASMR, only allows one or two products to be awarded Level I, and up to five products to be awarded Level II per annum. Most products are awarded Level III (15–20%), Level IV (around 50%) or Level V (around 30%) each year.

The Health Products Economic Committee

The Health Products Economic Committee becomes responsible for negotiating prices with companies and regulating drug expenditures at the global level once positive advice for reimbursement has been given.

This second step of the institutional framework involves a price negotiation with the company. This process, although it is far less formal than the previous step, is generally based on the following factors:

▶ clinical evaluation (i.e. ASMR level)

▶ market size

▶ prices in the top five European markets

▶ macro-economic objectives

▶ parallel exports threat.

In essence, the Health Products Economic Committee receives advice from the Minister of Health on the targets for the growth rate of healthcare expenditure and, more specifically, for pharmaceutical expenditure. Also, the parallel exports threat is taken into account and may result in a slightly higher price, in order to avoid or reduce parallel trade. The price negotiations will end up with a signed agreement on price, sales expectations, indications and further studies to be undertaken.

The Health Products Economic Committee set a very low target for growth in reimbursed medicines expenditure for 2006: 1%. This 1% growth rate target is similar to the growth rate in units (around 1%) and lower than the growth rate in value terms (5%) between 2004 and 2005. If the growth in pharmaceutical expenditure exceeds the target, companies have to pay back the difference, in accordance with a complicated scheme (the so-called 'convention') which defines individual contributions.

The Health Products Economic Committee examines about 1000 dossiers (presentations) per year, which involves around 500 new products. The average time for the whole reimbursement and pricing process is 243 days – one of the longest in Europe. For new products, the process takes even longer: 312 days (for 2002). If we break up the 312 days between the first and second stages (reimbursement and price decision, respectively), the Health Products Economic Committee, including price negotiation, is responsible for the greater part of the delay (173 days), leaving the Transparency Commission responsible for the remaining delay of 139 days. In addition, only 55% of new products are dealt with within the legal maximum six-month delay set out in the EU Transparency Directive.

The logic behind P&R in France

In a classic market approach, when the consumer makes a decision, he makes his own assessment of the product; the consumer observes the effectiveness, the price claimed, and makes a decision by balancing the benefit and the cost. To a certain extent, this is the approach used by the National Institute for Health and Clinical Excellence (NICE) in the UK, where the price, the cost and the effectiveness are compared and the prescribing recommendations are made on a cost per quality adjusted life-year (QALY) basis.

The French regulatory approach is somewhat different. The authorities observe effectiveness and take the decision to reimburse the drug (or not). Then they try to negotiate the lowest possible price for a given effectiveness. At no stage, therefore, do they balance effectiveness and price. The French scheme results in more products being evaluated and accepted but at a lower price as compared to the UK scheme, as the decision is based on effectiveness evidence alone. Figure 1.2 represents this system pictorially.

It would be interesting, from a theoretical point of view, to see when and where the two processes (i.e. the 'market approach' and the 'French regulatory' approach) may result in the same decisions. This may be the case on many occasions. However,

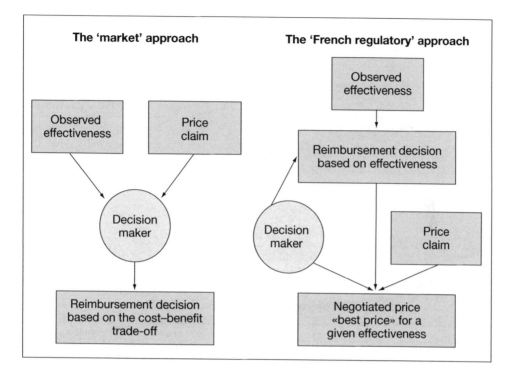

FIGURE 1.2   The 'market' versus the 'French regulatory' approach for decision making.

there may be sharp differences in pharmaceuticals bringing a little benefit to patients with severe diseases: the French approach grants reimbursement status to these drugs, although they may not be deemed cost-effective by NICE.

In this context, pharmaco-economic studies cannot be seen by authorities as an optimisation tool in a process of collective choice making, given that there is no trade-off between effectiveness and cost. Pharmaco-economic studies are seen more as a negotiation tool for companies to defend the price; it is not a tool in the hands of public authorities to make the most cost-effective decision in order to optimise public funds.

Recent changes in P&R regulation

There are many changes taking place in the French pharmaceutical market. I will focus on the changes related to the *Haute Autorité en Santé*, the Transparency Commission, the Health Products Economic Committee and the use of post-launch studies.

Haute Autorité en Santé

As mentioned before, a new evaluation institution, the *Haute Autorité en Santé* (HAS), has been created, at the beginning of 2005. It does not have a long history and therefore it is difficult to evaluate its actions so far. There is a board of eight experts and a large administrative body. The HAS is a single entity for medical evaluation, and now incorporates the three previous bodies that dealt with medical evaluation: the Transparency Commission; the Transparency Commission for Medical Devices (CEPP); and the Agency for Medical Technology Assessment (ANAES). The mission of HAS is to:

▶ have a global perspective in healthcare

▶ appraise all medical interventions (i.e. drugs, medical devices, medical procedures) for admission to reimbursement

▶ produce clinical guidelines for diagnosis and treatment

▶ accredit hospitals and professionals on the basis of quality standards.

In theory, it is a purely 'scientific' entity, which means 'economics' is not part of the process. Economic criteria do not play any official role in the HAS decision-making process. In practice, however, it can be the case that a device considered as 'expensive' will be treated in a different way from a non-expensive device, with a more demanding medical evaluation.

The Transparency Commission

The Transparency Commission has also been revised and given a new Chair, Professor Bouvenot. Medical expertise and public health issues have been reinforced, which means fewer clinicians and more epidemiologists are being involved. Also, new concepts have been introduced. For instance, the Commission will now evaluate the 'expected' medical service, rather than the 'rendered' medical service. As mentioned before, medical service is expected to be based on clinical trials rather than 'rendered' because, to be rendered, an effective medical service has to be evaluated according to real-life data. Drugs therefore have to conform to expectations based on real-life evaluation.

A new evaluation criterion has been included: 'public health interest'. It is not founded on law but rather on the practice of the Commission. This new criterion takes into account:

▶ severity of the disease

▶ 'quantity of effect', that is, the magnitude of any positive difference

▶ effectiveness/side effect profile

▶ the impact of the healthcare system as a whole (e.g. the substitution to outpatient care from inpatient care)

▶ the impact on the population's health (e.g. existence of an uncovered need or the existence of reliable criteria to define the target population).

The last criterion is a very important one, and basically tries to answer the following questions.

▶ Is it possible to have very precise criteria to define who is eligible for the drug?

▶ Are there any tools to identify the right patients?

Another aspect of the 'public health interest' factor is the interaction between the use of medicines and other health-related segments. For instance, a drug may take a patient out of hospital or facilitate outpatient treatment. This would be an additional benefit.

The 'public health interest' is evaluated separately and takes into account the effect on the healthcare system of using the health technology which is being evaluated. It is a population approach rather than a patient approach, and is consistent with the trend in France that public health specialists are gradually having more influence, at the expense of other clinicians.

Price Committee

There is also a new Price Committee in France. As mentioned before, it used to be a committee of civil servants; now it is composed of a mix of civil servants, three representatives of the public health funds and one representative of the complementary private health insurance funds. In other words, the input of payers has been strengthened.

There have been two innovations in the process of the Price Committee. First, a price notification procedure has been set up to speed up the pricing procedure, although it is limited to some innovative products and to hospital-regulated products. Companies have to inform the Price Committee about the price the company is planning to charge for their product; this price will be accepted within 15 days provided that the:

▶ price is consistent with the price in the top-five European markets

- price is consistent with the prices of equivalent drugs
- company has provided sales forecasts originating from the medicine's licensed indication.

The second new element in the pricing process is the new two-tier pricing approach, which applies in certain special circumstances; namely, when products are under threat from extensive parallel trade. If this is the case, the price is divided between a nominal market price and a real price after rebate which is paid annually to the health insurance funds. However, it is not very transparent, as the size of rebates is not publicly available. It may introduce some distortion, because the observed market price is not the real price, and the real price is not known publicly.

Post-launch studies

Post-launch studies are part of the agreement between the government and the pharmaceutical industry for the period 2003–2006. The agreement states that 'the parties agree about the need to produce data on the effects of the use of new pharmaceuticals in real life' (LEEM, 2004). For instance, the expected 'public health interest' discussed above will need to be confirmed by appropriate post-launch studies.

Post-launch studies mainly concern pharmaceuticals that:

- are targeted at a very large population
- may be prescribed outside their labelled indications
- are likely to have a significant effect on healthcare organisations.

The post-launch studies should preferably use health insurance claims data. The problem is that health insurers do not yet collaborate too much in this process, because of lack of time and expertise. Companies have still to carry out these post-launch studies and produce their own data with specific surveys and questionnaires. The protocol, the scientific committee and the methodology used for these post-launch studies have to be agreed by the Transparency Committee. The agreement also states that the cost must remain reasonable, although there is no definition of what is deemed as 'reasonable'.

Although some large scale post-launch studies were undertaken (for instance the CADEUS study on the use of Cox-2 inhibitors, commissioned by the Health Products Economic Committee, and undertaken by the Epidemiology and Public

Health Department of Bordeaux University) there remains a need for clarification of methodological issues as well as 'political' consequences: how the results of such studies can affect the pricing and reimbursement process is not fully clear.

National P&R policies in the future

Sustainability of the French healthcare system

Forecasting the future is always a difficult task. While the French healthcare system is in deep deficit, of around €10 billion per year (deficits in 2004 and 2005 totalled €11.7 billion and €9.7 billion, respectively, and the forecasted deficit for 2006 amounts to €7 billion), the government is optimistically planning to reach a financial equilibrium by 2009.

The deficit is currently financed by the debt. By June 2005, the health insurance debt was more than €100 billion, which represents 10% of the total public debt (about €1000 billion). The government has excluded the option of raising health insurance revenue. Let us recall that the French health insurance is financed by payroll taxes up to 60%, and by taxation – a special income tax – up to 40%. The introduction of this income tax in 1990, called Contribution Social Généralisée (CSG), marked a departure from the strict 'Bismarckian' model where insurance is a fringe benefit from employment and where healthcare is financed jointly by employers and employees. In fact CSG is paid by everybody, irrespective of their professional status. Raising the flat CSG rate from 7.5%, the current percentage, to 8.5% would yield about €8 billion per year, thus covering the current deficit. However, in the presence of fiscal competition among countries, France's tax rates are already high in comparison with other countries. The situation is, therefore, very challenging at the present, with a deep deficit, an important debt, high tax rates and a slow economic growth!

New reforms

Facing this situation the choice of the government was to maintain the basic characteristics of the systems – excluding thus any 'big bang reform' – and to look for productivity gains which may result from a better organisation and a stricter management of the system.

This was the philosophy of the reform voted by the Parliament in August 2004. The most spectacular measures were the adoption of a 'soft' gate-keeping system under which direct access to specialised care is still possible, although it will be made more expensive for patients, and the introduction of mandatory computerised medical records to help doctors make appropriate decisions. Hospital financing was modified, passing from global budget to a more modern DRG system. Quality controls are more systematically performed. The overall healthcare management capacity was improved with a reinforced power of the general manager of the public insurance fund.

However, this is a long-term reform and in the short term the government has tried to generate some savings. An agreement was reached with the pharmaceutical industry to save €2.1 billion for the period 2002–2007. In November 2005, however, the government implemented other measures to try to save an additional €1 billion in 2006. These measures include:

▶ introducing a special tax, equivalent to 1.76% of turnover

▶ reference pricing for drugs with a low generic penetration rate

▶ de-reimbursement of some drugs deemed to represent 'low therapeutic value'.

On the demand side, the new 'convention' signed with medical unions aimed to generate savings on prescriptions of up to €1 billion in 2005 and, in particular, savings from prescriptions of statins, hypnotics and antibiotics, plus sick leave prescriptions. Nevertheless, the large part of this €1 billion saving will necessarily come from medicines' expenditure. Table 1.1 shows the (expected) cumulative savings in pharmaceutical expenditure as a result of the 2005–2007 agreement for prescriptions drugs.

TABLE 1.1 Cumulative savings in pharmaceutical expenditure, 2005–2007 (€ million)

	2005	2006	2007
Generic drugs	330	700	1050
'Big boxes' (3-month treatment)	80	130	180
Negotiated price cuts	100	200	350
Hospital drugs regulation	50	80	100
Fiscal measures	180	180	180
De-reimbursement	50	150	250
Total	790	1440	2110

What are the expectations?

To some extent, we face an unprecedented situation in France. Healthcare expenditure is growing slowly, at around 2.5% to 3.5%, and it is difficult to imagine the healthcare system growing at a lower rate than that. But despite the slow growth, the deficit is huge. As general economic growth is even slower than the growth rate of healthcare expenditure, the deficit will certainly be maintained and perhaps even increased.

The official position which focuses mainly or exclusively on the improvement of the system management is correct but insufficient. In my opinion, it is important to draw attention to the financing side of the problem, which implies:

▶ extending private out-of-pocket payments, such as deductibles and co-payments

▶ changing public financing patterns by switching the remaining payroll taxes to general taxation, which is less harmful to employment; this policy can also bring additional revenue and decrease the cost of labour.

However, this reform will be very difficult, given that any change in the healthcare system needs to have a minimal effect on consumers. So far, the scope of the reform has related to healthcare professionals and health insurance firms. Patients do not pay for much of their care, given that most of the care is delivered at present without any co-payments. Given the situation and the trends in healthcare, it seems difficult to imagine that consumers can still benefit for long from the very large 'drawing right' they have been accustomed to.

Such a change is politically difficult and costly. France is entering an election period – a new president will be elected in spring 2007 – which is not favourable to dramatic changes. Therefore the future remains uncertain. Regarding the pharmaceutical industry, however, no changes should be expected in terms of pricing and reimbursement policy in the next two years.

Discussion

The use of cost-effectiveness evidence in P&R procedures – the economic component of post-launch studies

Q: Are health outcomes and cost-effectiveness becoming more or less important? You seem to imply that the economic part is becoming less important but, on the other hand, there are the post-launch studies you mentioned. I am unclear how significant the economic component of those will be.

A: The mentality of people, especially in the administration or in the medical profession, is to consider economics outside of this. Economics is just price and negotiation. The 'noble' part of the job is to evaluate the drugs medically. After that, you just negotiate the price on the back of the results obtained from the clinical evaluation.

Post-launch studies follow that ideology. In fact, they more or less replace a cost-effectiveness study, but without the economics, that is, without the cost. The post-launch studies are simply to document the pattern of use. They are of interest for a number of reasons: you can have outcome research studies; you can enlarge study endpoints; you can make quality-of-life assessments; and you can give a better view of the real effectiveness of the drug.

Generally speaking, we add a pharmaco-economic level to these studies, but it is just an add-on; it is not officially taken into account. Pharmaco-economics influences decision-making but it is not an official criterion on which to base a decision.

Collaborations between European health bodies

Q: You have commented on the workload of reviews that the agencies need to do. Do you see any tendency for collaboration between the French authorities and the other European countries' authorities, or with a pan-European authority? What is your assessment of the current political intentions there?

A: With NICE in the UK, the HAS in France and now the Institute for Quality and Efficiency in Healthcare (IQWiG) in Germany there is clearly a trend towards a reinforcement of medical – and economic – evaluation of medical technologies. I think that there will shortly be a meeting between the main Chairs of the IQWiG, HAS and NICE. The methodologies, processes and missions of these three agencies are different, but I believe they want to exchange information and observations.

Parallel trade

Q: You mentioned that the new Health Products Economic Committee will, in a sense, look at G10, recommendation 6-type arrangements – a nominal price and a rebate, that is, the separation of the reimbursement price from the market price – for certain drugs which meet certain criteria. Earlier, you implied that the number of drugs which would be able to benefit from that would be very small. Could you comment on that?

A: The French authorities have always said that this kind of arrangement (the two-tier pricing system and the new approach of the European Commission – G10, recommendation 6) cannot be part of a regulated system. It is simply to manage a few cases on a case-by-case basis. It is not designed to replace the usual system of direct price regulation. This point is very clearly stated.

Patient co-payment

Q: You mentioned that there was a prospect of new policy around patient co-payment, which at present is very low. Is there any real political interest in pursuing that idea?

A: My feeling is that we are slowly changing the philosophy of the French healthcare system. The tendency – although there is not full consciousness of it – is that we cover up to 100%, with an exhaustive package of services and no restriction on access to care. My feeling is that eventually we will have catastrophic insurance – paying 100% for severe disease – and large co-payment and private health insurance for the rest of the pathology. There is a move towards this kind of separation.

For instance, at present for about eight million people – 20% of the adult population – there is no co-payment at all; they are reimbursed 100% for all care, because they have a severe condition. This group is expanding, and one million people a year enter this system. Thus, there are many exceptions to the co-payment, including co-payments for pregnant women. At the same time, the government has raised the deductible for some surgical procedures.

There are two tendencies. On the one hand, they de-reimburse some drugs of low therapeutic value and extend public coverage for people with severe conditions; on the other, they increase co-payments and the participation of the consumer in the financing of some services. The two policies are not contradictory. It is a dual system. It is full coverage by catastrophic public health insurance, and another type of insurance for non-catastrophic conditions, dominated either by the private insurance system or by direct payments from the consumer (i.e. self-insurance).

Rebates and innovative drugs

Q: Regarding the expenditure caps on pharmaceuticals both at the global level and for individual companies, how does innovation get factored into those?

A: Innovation is not included in the cap. The cap is for the total of drug expenditure but, when you compute the contribution of each company, there is a complicated formula which takes into account the growth rate of sales, promotional expenditure and so on. In that formula, innovative drugs are excluded from the computation, so sales from innovative drugs are not included for rebate purposes.

The problem is that an innovative drug is an innovation for one year or two years. After this period, it joins the 'normal' drugs and is eligible for the cap and rebate system.

Companies argue that the expenditure cap is terrible for innovation and for the attractiveness of France, so foreign investment is leaving. The government has counter-arguments and shows examples of investments by foreign companies, such as Lilly and Novartis. France is a large market and companies are still investing. There is therefore an ongoing debate, where everyone is to some extent right and to some extent wrong.

Institutional framework and the development of a national pharmaceutical industry

Q: How does the French government encourage a healthy national pharmaceutical industry?

A: It is against European law so there are no formal measures to encourage it. French companies are closer to the decision-makers; they have a close relationship and they know how to use the system. This is more to do with the power of influence. I guess that it is the same in many countries; some companies are better treated than others, not officially but effectively.

The level of prices, the constraints in terms of whether or not supplementary studies have to be carried out, whether the study is large or small and so on, are all details which can give a feeling that one group of companies is treated better than the other. The relationship between the public and the private sector is partly based on official rules and partly on informal relationships.

Generics penetration in France

Q: The government has been trying to encourage generics. Has it been successful?

A: In the last 10 years some efforts have been made to promote a generics market. First – in the early 1990s – there was an attempt to create a generic products supply. At that time generic drugs did not have a significant presence in the market. Some companies were encouraged to develop a supply of generic products, with the possibility of getting better prices for their innovative products as a counterpart. This first attempt was a failure, as a supply without a demand does not create a market. The second step dates back to 1999, when pharmacists were allowed to substitute generics and the margin system was changed. The market started to grow at that time. The real take-off took place in 2002 when doctors' fees were raised subject to the condition that they encourage the use of generics. Competition among generics manufacturers has also played a positive role, as they have offered better financial conditions to pharmacists. Pharmacists' margins are in fact higher for generics than for the corresponding original molecule. Currently the substitution rate is about 60% in units and 50% in value and it keeps rising.

Paradoxically, the government has introduced a reference price system for some products where branded original molecules are reimbursed on the basis of generic prices and the patient has to pay the difference, if the price of the branded product is higher than the generic's. Within this system, companies tend to align prices and incentives for pharmacists disappear, as the margins of original products and generics tend to be the same. The government does not really understand how incentives work in the pharmaceutical market. It wants both generics and reference pricing but it is not aware of the fact that this can be contradictory.

Reference

Les enterprises du médicament (LEEM) (2004) Accord-cadre 2003–2006.

CHAPTER 2

Pricing and reimbursement policies in Germany: current and future trends

J-Matthias Graf von der Schulenburg

The aim of this chapter is to describe the German pricing and reimbursement system. In order to do this, however, there is a need to analyse the current general situation in Germany, and in particular, the situation of the healthcare system. The idea is thus to discuss the pricing and reimbursement of pharmaceuticals in Germany within a broader framework, by taking into account what is the current, and what could be the future, situation of the German social security and healthcare systems.

Overview of the healthcare system in Germany

To begin, we will analyse the financial contributions made to social security providers in Germany; that is, nursing insurance (which is relatively new), unemployment insurance, sickness funds (Germany's social health insurance) and the pension funds. Expressed as a percentage of income, Figure 2.1 shows some model

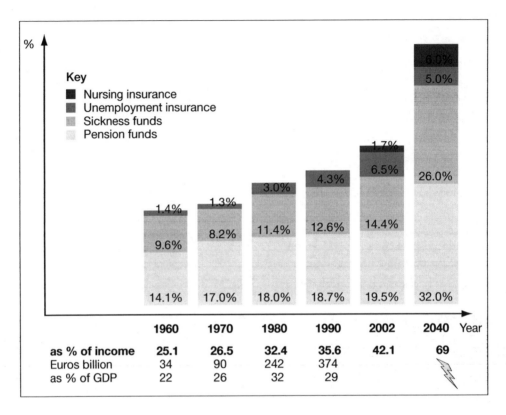

FIGURE 2.1   Contributions to social security as percentage of income.

calculations of these various contribution rates to social security providers over a specific period of time. The figures relate to the period starting in 1960, and show how these contributions would evolve up to and including 2040 if no reforms of the social security system were implemented. In Germany, the contribution to social security providers is paid by employers and employees from their income. Figure 2.1 shows the contributions in 1960 (25.1% of income), which rose to 42.1% in 2002 and would, if there were no reforms, increase to 69% by 2040. This means that the 'tsunami' of the baby-boomer generation – those born in the 1960s – would sweep away all of the social security schemes if nothing were to be done about the income, the financing and, of course, the expenditure.

Looking at this framework, it is clear that the government in Germany will be trying to control these contributions, so that contributions for sickness funds do not increase from the current 14% of income to about 26% by 2040, which is what the projections in Figure 2.1 illustrate.

An acceptance of rate of contribution increases to the extent outlined above is not conceivable. That would mean an 'explosive device' for the financing of the social security systems and over the increase of the ancillary wages would imply that the international competitive ability of German enterprises will be endangered.

Broadly speaking, there are two forms of health service internationally.

▶ National health services, mainly financed by taxes (like in the UK).

▶ Social health insurance schemes (Bismarckian schemes), such as the German one, mainly financed by contributions.

In addition, in Germany there are social aid systems with special programmes for particular groups of society. This system is not a general healthcare system. Here you define, for instance, different population segments according to a number of criteria such as income level, age, gender, number of dependent children, for whom special programmes are designed and put into place.

The challenge for health insurance schemes such as the German one is that contributions are taken mainly from the employers, which means that if these contributions rise, it can cause unemployment. Contributions are also taken from those who are insured. This includes only those who are commercially employed but not the self-employed or civil servants. The challenge is how to find other sources of finance for these healthcare systems and, in particular, to decide whether the system becomes more tax-financed. A change to greater tax funding of healthcare would mean the government taking steps to introduce greater regulation of the market than at the present time. The reason for this is that once the State is paying for something it also wants to control it. This rationale also applies to the pharmaceutical market.

The Bismarckian system in Germany is based on a law passed in 1883 which established the social security scheme. This law only had five pages and regulated the system for 50 years. Nowadays, there are about 6000 laws regulating the German system. The question is whether or not the Bismarckian model will remain in place. Of course, any change in the healthcare system will obviously have a big impact on the future pharmaceutical pricing and reimbursement system in Germany.

In 2003 Germany was the fourth-highest country in terms of per capita healthcare spending, behind the US, Switzerland and Norway. Healthcare expenditure is increasing around the world, and certainly in Germany.

So what are the main characteristics of the German healthcare system? First, healthcare expenditures represent around 10% of gross national product (GNP). Second, there are 280 sickness funds, which is a significant decrease from the 1200 that existed 20 years ago. A big consolidation process among the sickness funds has been taking place. This means that healthcare providers are facing increasing monopoly power on the other side of the market, where there are now a few conglomerate sickness funds negotiating with the payers, with greater market power than in the past.

Third, the doctors' insurance associations are very dominant. There are 23 regional doctors' insurance associations. Currently they continue to regulate the ambulatory care market. The associations also have a great influence on the prescription behaviour of physicians in ambulatory care, because they set their budgets. Whether or not this power should remain in place has been discussed by every government over the last 20 years, but no government has succeeded in breaking their power.

It is also important to mention that Germany's current general economic situation is characterised by a low gross domestic product (GDP) growth rate and a high unemployment rate, coupled with severe structural problems. Innovations in financing, providing and reimbursing healthcare services are indispensable for cost-effective health insurance and healthcare provision that meet the needs of the population.

Overview of the German pharmaceutical market

In line with the increase in healthcare expenditure seen in Germany, expenditure on pharmaceuticals has also increased in recent years. For instance, pharmaceutical expenditure grew by 14% in 2004, which is quite high and poses a challenge for health policy to do something about it.

Current trends in national P&R regulation

Let us first discuss the P&R mechanisms directed towards the patient and the physician. Germany's social health insurance (SHI) system provides prescription pharmaceuticals as an in-kind benefit to the insured. Patients must only pay legally defined co-payments, which represent the difference between the market price and reference price of a prescription pharmaceutical and are equal to 10% of the price, with a minimum of €5 and a maximum of €10. Out-of-pocket payments have increased over the last few years.

There is a reference price system, and any difference between the market price and the reference price becomes effectively a compulsory co-payment if the more expensive product is dispensed. In fact, Germany was the first country to introduce such a system with the Healthcare Reform Act of 1989. The reference price scheme is relatively straightforward. There are three groups – 1, 2 and 3 – and the last two include drugs still under patent. The reference price system has been implemented in four stages, in 1989, 1991, 1992 and 2004, and by 1997 it covered 60% of the pharmaceutical market. There are still some difficulties with respect to the calculation of the reference prices.

Office-based physicians (i.e. those providing ambulatory care) have individual drug budgets. If the drug budget is exceeded, the physician has to explain the excess, which implies filling in a large number of forms. The act of filling in forms is obviously disliked, and hence physicians do not usually exceed their drug budgets.

We now turn to price regulation. The standard official comment is to say 'There is no price regulation in Germany. The pharmaceutical industry is totally free to set whatever prices it wants.' However, there is price regulation in Germany and an increasing number of measures to control prices have been introduced over the past decades, including:

- fixed dispensing fees for pharmacies of €8.10 per pack of prescription-only medicines plus a fixed margin of 3% of the wholesale price

- the reference price system, which is an indirect price control, covering both off-patent and in-patent medicines

- a €2 pharmacy rebate per prescription-only drug plus a further 6% 'tax' (patented drugs) and a 10% tax (non-patented drugs) for pharmaceutical producers in the form of rebates on the prices paid for non-reference-priced medicines bought by the statutory sickness funds.

In addition, new institutions have been created which might influence the price and reimbursement system in Germany, for instance, the Institute for Quality and Efficiency in Medical Care (IQWiG), created in 2004, which is sometimes called 'the German NICE'.* However, this is the wrong term to use because, among other differences, the IQWiG is not structured in the same way as NICE. The role played by this new institute in terms of health technology assessment is discussed later.

There are also new reimbursement schemes which influence medicine prices. The DRG system in the hospital market in Germany will have a big influence

---

* NICE, the National Institute for Health and Clinical Excellence, *see* Chapter 3 for more information on this organisation.

on how much hospitals will pay for pharmaceuticals in the future, because the hospitals receive a reference price from the sickness funds for each case they treat. There are also higher patient co-payment rates and, for pharmaceuticals, the so-called 'fourth hurdle' – the health technology assessment programmes. They are used to evaluate the efficacy, effectiveness, comparative effectiveness, efficiency, and the social, legal and ethical implications of healthcare.

Additionally, there are integrated treatment programmes and disease management programmes in Germany. The rationale of those programmes is that, ultimately, providers will negotiate with the suppliers, and in particular with the pharmaceutical industry, how medicines will be provided, in what quantity and at what price.

Recent changes in P&R regulation

Changes within the overall healthcare system

Before discussing the changes in the German pharmaceutical market in particular, first, we need to address some changes that have taken place in the overall healthcare system. In this respect, Germany is taking the same route as other countries in three ways. First, Germany is to set up more and more agencies or institutions; second, structural changes are being made; and third, there is increased transparency and integration of the healthcare system.

In terms of institutions and commissions, there are three of particular note in Germany. First, there is the Statistical Office for Medical Treatment (DIMDI), which provides health technology assessment studies. DIMDI collaborates with different preferred provider institutes in Germany which perform such studies and two of these are based in Hanover – one at the medical school and one at the university. Second, there is the IQWiG. However, it is still early days to explain the exact route the IQWiG is following. What we have seen, however, is that DIMDI and the IQWiG are somewhat in competition. The IQWiG is paying higher prices than DIMDI for carrying out health technology assessment studies. This implies there is competition between government agencies. The third and most powerful agency is the Joint Federal Committee – *Gemeinsamer Bundesausschuss* (GBA). This institution makes decisions about the sickness fund system, defines the guidelines for the determination of groups of pharmaceuticals that are subject to the reference price scheme, determines reference price groups, which drugs will be included in the benefit schedule and which treatment guidelines will be laid down.

The other issue where Germany is following other countries closely is regarding structural changes. Germany's social health insurance system has undergone a number of extensive reforms over the past decades and there will be large structural changes in Germany in the years to come. Eventually compulsory insurance will cover the entire population, in order to obtain more resources for the statutory healthcare system. The issue of how to finance the German healthcare system still needs to be resolved. The discussion focuses on whether the system should be financed by higher taxes or whether Germany should remain with the present contribution-financed healthcare scheme. Currently, in Germany, we can also see the beginnings of public–private partnerships, that is, public and private institutions working together. With the sickness funds, public sickness funds work together with private health insurers, and the same applies in the hospital sector. For instance, Hamburg has sold its public hospitals to a private hospital chain, and they manage the hospitals together.

There is also the matter of transparency and patient rights. Patient rights play a big role in the European Union (EU) context. Every country is required to have a patient representative in their commissions. In the joint federal commission there is a patient representative, who already has a big influence and who will have an increasing influence in the future. For the pharmaceutical industry in the future, as with all other healthcare suppliers in our system, patients will play a much more important role than they have in the past. On the other hand, the role played by opinion-formers, who were the target of marketing in the past, will become less important.

Finally, what can we say about the effects of the coalition treaty between the Christian Democratic Union (CDU) and Social Democratic Party (SPD) of November 2005 for Germany's healthcare system? Not much; there is very little in the treaty about health, and discussion of the healthcare system has been postponed to 2007.

Medicines' market

Concerning medicines in particular, the government has announced a number of new regulations. For instance, non-monetary rebates given to pharmacists by pharmaceutical companies will be banned in the future. There will be a 5% price decrease for generics, and it seems that the physicians' responsibility with respect to drugs will be strengthened. This strengthening could imply physicians facing much tighter drug budgets. Physicians would then examine with greater care what they prescribe and how much it costs. In addition, a price freeze has been enforced for two years. This compulsory price freeze is definitely against the German constitution, but given that any probable litigation against this price freeze will take at least two years, the enforced price freeze will still go ahead.

The government has also said that it wants to distinguish between 'real' and 'fake' innovations. This distinction can become a vital one, given it is the issue which arises in defining the German reference price system for drugs under patent. Thus, two important questions arise.

▶ How can a drug show additional benefits compared with those drugs that are already on the market?

▶ Are those additional benefits – for instance, better compliance by patients because the drug has to be taken only once a day rather than twice – significant enough that the new medicine can be considered an innovation?

Under the new rules of Germany's reference price system, which were introduced in January 2004, a single reference price can be defined for a group that includes patented as well as non-patented products (so-called 'Jumbo-Groups'). The new regulation allows for the exclusion from reference price regulations of patented products with significant additional therapeutic benefits or fewer side effects than other drugs. The Joint Federal Committee is responsible for determining whether a significant additional therapeutic benefit or fewer side effects is given. Since the law does not define what is meant by 'significant additional benefit', the Joint Federal Committee has considerable freedom in its decision to include innovative drugs in a reference price group. Although all decision makers in Germany's healthcare system agree that innovation is necessary for the advancement of the healthcare system, political debate focuses largely on the discussion of 'fake' innovations. Application of the reference price system to patented pharmaceuticals was meant to make a distinction between important and trivial innovations. This would require the establishment of an independent institution that is able to determine the value of innovations from a societal perspective. The Joint Federal Committee, which is made up of representatives of office-based physicians, SHI funds and hospitals, is not appropriate for this task.

The use of health technology assessments in Germany

We now focus attention on the use of health technology assessments (HTA), which has been reinforced in Germany with the foundation of the IQWiG. Since 1990, the systematic use of HTA as a tool for the evaluation of all medical procedures has increased considerably in Europe. Studies are carried out on both medicines and other health technologies or services. The process starts with the collection of all the available information on medical effectiveness, the economic consequences, the legal consequences and ethical aspects of the medical service in question. Once all this information is collected, judgements are made about how good and reliable this information is.

What has been the evolution of HTA in Germany over the last years? The German government announced its first HTA assessment in 1995. In 2001, DIMDI became the official organiser of Germany's HTA programme. In the future, responsibility for the HTA programme will rest either with DIMDI or the IQWiG, or both. Until now it has not been made clear which institution will be responsible for this programme. The HTA studies that have been carried out in Germany may be found on the DIMDI website (www.dimdi.de).

The IQWiG was created in 2004 with the following responsibilities:

▶ provision of information for patients

▶ elaboration of evidence-based guidelines

▶ elaboration of scientific HTA studies in co-operation with the German Institute for Medical Documentation

▶ elaboration of guidelines for drug therapy and reference prices.

The IQWiG has set down how it would like to carry out the HTA studies. Unfortunately, it has not stuck to its own stated methods, as was pointed out in a recent article where the first HTA study on statins was discussed (Kulp *et al.*, 2005). However, these studies will play a dominant role in the future in terms of how pricing and reimbursement of pharmaceuticals is carried out in Germany, and in Europe more widely.

National P&R policies in the future

This section offers some views as to what the future could hold for Germany's pharmaceutical market. Before discussing what may be the two most important issues for the future, consider some general remarks. The administration of sickness funds in Germany – which in the past were relatively simple organisations that just took money in and gave money out – is getting smarter, and they are learning from each other and from other countries. This implies a need to look at the global picture to see what other governments around the world are doing. We may expect that all the good ideas will be taken up by the administration in our own country.

A more sophisticated reference price system will end up covering almost all of the pharmaceutical market. In addition, healthcare systems will become more integrated, whereby there will be global payments for the treatment of certain diseases. This integration will create more pressure on those agents who provide services in those systems and, in turn, greater pressure on pharmaceutical products.

Now, let us focus on two important dimensions that will drive the future of the German pharmaceutical market. First, the possibility of rationing healthcare provision, and how this will be implemented; second, the future role of economic evaluation in Germany, and whether evaluations will be done in commissions behind closed doors, or in a more transparent manner.

Rationing and provision of healthcare

There are a number of international studies that examine whether or not rationing is taking place, and in what countries. For instance, a recent publication tries to understand how the general population, decision-makers and professionals in medical care in six countries (Finland, France, Germany, Portugal, Spain and the UK) would like their healthcare system to be in the future (Graf von der Schulenburg and Blanke, 2004). In order to do this, a European empirical study was put together which asked these three stakeholder groups about their views. All these stakeholder groups were questioned because it was thought they play an important role in our society. In addition, it is not only what politicians want to do and what regulations they enforce, but also what other interest groups really want.

So, what does the general population want? Table 2.1 shows, among other things, what the general population thinks about how the healthcare system should be financed. For instance, in Germany, a minority (28%) says that it should be funded by taxation; or, in other words, the large majority (72%) say 'no' to the option of funding the system mainly by taxes. This is different from the UK, where 86% of the general population think their healthcare system should be tax-funded.

Regarding whether or not healthcare expenditure should be limited, and again referring to Table 2.1, the majority of the population (63%) in Germany say 'no'. The majority also say 'no' to the possibility of taxes being used to create a more generous healthcare system. On the other hand, Germans do not want an increase in premiums for a more generous health system, but in most countries – with the exception of France – they are probably more willing to pay out of pocket expenses (i.e. user charges). I think this is a message which we should publicise more than we have done in the past.

TABLE 2.1 General population: money, from where?

	Finland	France	Germany	Portual	Spain	UK
Financing by taxation	69%	47%	28%	59%	59%	86%
Expenditure should be limited	28%	51%	37%	28%	23%	42%
Higher taxes for a more generous health system	36%	29%	24%	37%	59%	67%
Higher premiums for a more generous health system	50%	29%	42%	22%	46%	38%
Reaction to paying user charges in order to obtain a reduction in premium	Positive	Negative	Postive	Positive	Even	Even

Source: Graf von der Schulenburg and Blanke (2004).

Table 2.2 shows the results obtained when the general population was asked whether or not they had experienced rationing, and if so, in what health sector.

TABLE 2.2 General population: have you experienced rationing in healthcare?

	Finland	France	Germany	Portugal	Spain	UK
Percentage having been affected in the past	24	62	28	85	14	21
If affected, which sector:						
particular treatment withheld	87%	49%	41%	NA	38%	51%
particular medication not prescribed	13%	20%	55%	NA	50%	20%
Other	0%	31%	4%	NA	12%	29%

NA, not available

Source: Graf von der Schulenburg and Blanke (2004).

TABLE 2.3 Professionals: how can we save money?

Ranking	Finland	France	Germany	Portugal	Spain	UK
1	Generic pharmaceuticals	Clinical guidelines	Co-insurance	Positive list for pharmaceuticals	Positive list for pharmaceuticals	Generic pharmaceuticals
2	Clinical guidelines	Co-insurance	Generic pharmaceuticals	Service provider budgets	Generic pharmaceuticals	Clinical guidelines
3	Positive list for pharmaceuticals	Generic pharmaceuticals	Clinical guidelines	Co-insurance	Clinical guidelines	Positive list for pharmaceuticals
4	Negative list for pharmaceuticals	Positive list for pharmaceuticals	Positive list for pharmaceuticals	Clinical guidelines	Service provider budgets	Negative list for pharmaceuticals
5	Co-insurance	Negative list for pharmaceuticals	Negative list for pharmaceuticals	Generic pharmaceuticals	Negative list for pharmaceuticals	Service provider budgets
6	Waiting lists	Service provider budgets	Service provider budgets	Negative list for pharmaceuticals	Co-insurance	Co-insurance
7	Service provider budgets	Waiting lists	Waiting lists	Waiting lists	Waiting lists	Waiting lists

Source: Graf von der Schulenburg and Blanke (2004).

In Germany, a minority of the interviewees (28%) from the 'general population' segment replied that until now, they had experienced rationing when treated. Of those who felt they had experienced rationing, 55% felt they had experienced it in relation to medicines, by not being treated with the most innovative drugs on the market. On the other hand, the results show that the majority of Portuguese (85%) felt they had been affected by rationing, while only 14% and 21% of Spanish and UK citizens, respectively, felt this way. Rationing of costly, new pharmaceutical products and medical technologies is one of the major objectives of current health policy. This is reality in most European countries and in particular in Germany.

When medical professionals were asked about the areas of healthcare where additional savings could be realised, in three (France, Portugal and the UK) out of the six countries, 'pharmaceuticals' represented the most prominent means of getting more money to finance the healthcare system. In Germany, however, 'the administration' comes first, followed by 'pharmaceuticals'. This result may have some policy implications for pharmaceuticals in the future: they may become the target of health policy, increasing the regulatory burden in this segment.

Table 2.3 illustrates the ranking of options in the six countries when professionals were asked 'How can we save money?' In most countries, policies related to pharmaceuticals (including generic medicines and positive lists) were usually in the top positions. In Germany, interestingly, co-insurance is the single most preferred option.

Role of economic evaluations

The second element regarding the way forward is the role that economic evaluations will play in Germany in the future. In terms of economic evaluation, the website www.euronheed.org offers interesting information. This is a new website which contains a collection of economic evaluation studies from around the world. It is financed by the EU, and the University of Hanover is carrying out the work for the German-speaking part. It gives a rating of the economic evaluation studies as to reliability. Data sources similar to this one will play a much bigger role in the future than they have in the past.

Related to economic evaluations are the elements of price and quantity (volume) control. A number of studies have been carried out on pricing and reimbursement trends in Europe (Graf von der Schulenburg, 2000; Eberhardt *et al.*, 2004). In particular, in the study by Eberhardt *et al.* under the name 'EUROMET (*European Network of Methodology and Application of Economic Evaluation Techniques*),

TABLE 2.4 Influence of economic evaluations in healthcare decision-making: a summary of EUROMET 2004

	France	Germany	UK	Italy	Norway	Spain	Sweden	Netherlands
Institutional requirements of economic evaluation studies (e.g. NICE, commissions and other expert groups)	+	–	+	+	+	+	+	+
Existence and design of *positive/negative lists*	+	+	+	+	+	Not explicitly mentioned	/	–
Influence of economic evaluation studies on *health policy process*	+	/	+	/	Not explicitly mentioned	+ (Extent of influence not explicitly mentioned)	/	+ (More indirectly)
Use of economic evaluation studies for *old products/patent products and innovative products*	/	–	+ (Stress is on innovative products)	/	/	Not at all – less	/	/
Influence of economic evaluation studies on *pricing and reimbursement* of drugs/medical devices	+ (Studies are a part of contract with the industry)	/	– (Influence is through NICE guidance)	+ (Studies are supporting)	+ (Studies are supporting)	+ (Little)	+ (Studies are supporting)	+ (Studies are supporting)
Influence of economic evaluation studies on *prescription patterns and treatment guidelines*	/	/	+ (Impact of guidance is uncertain)	+		+	+	+
Key players in decision making	+	+	+	+	+	+	+	+

	France	Germany	UK	Italy	Norway	Spain	Sweden	Netherlands
Distribution of knowledge of economic evaluation studies at different levels of decision making	Not explicitly mentioned	+	+ (Less knowledge, lower levels)	Not explicitly mentioned	+	+	+	Not explicitly mentioned
Existence of *governmental HTA*	+	+	+	–	+	+	+	+
Influence of economic evaluations for *health programmes* (e.g. disease management programmes)	/	–	/	/	/	–	/	/
Informal and formal requirements and guidelines for economic evaluation studies at *present and in future*	/	+	+ (Formal NICE guidelines)	–	+	+ (Informal)	Not explicitly mentioned	+

+ = Existent; – = Non-existent; / = Not mentioned.

NICE, National Institute for Health and Clinical Excellence; HTA, health technology assessments.

Source: Eberhardt *et al.* (2004).

how economic evaluation studies influence healthcare decision-makers in various countries was analysed. France, Germany, the Netherlands, Norway, Spain and the UK participated in both EUROMET 2000 and EUROMET 2004. Austria, Finland and Portugal were involved only in the 2000 study, while Italy and Sweden participated only in the 2004 study.

Table 2.4, which relates to the 2004 publication, illustrates how economic evaluations influence healthcare decision-making in eight European countries. For instance, and focusing on Germany, results show that at the time of publication of EUROMET 2004 there were no institutional requirements for economic evaluation studies. On the other hand, economic evaluation studies have some influence on the existence and design of positive/negative lists. Another interesting result for Germany is that there is no explicit mention of the influence of economic evaluation studies on the health policy process.

As a final comment, Table 2.4 shows there is no clear trend in Europe as to the influence of economic evaluation studies on healthcare decision-making. While it is clear that economic evaluation will start to play a more prominent role in the future, it will be interesting to see how exactly this influence is manifested.

Discussion

Industrial policy and the pharmaceutical industry

Q: I think that the German pharmaceutical industry is presently playing in the second league. The industry has lost a great deal of market share and influence in the last 20 years. Do you see any measures, incentives or configurations on the part of politicians to end this trend, and to do something for the local industry?

A: No. German health policy is not industrial policy. These tasks are separated in government and will remain like this in the future.

However, I should perhaps give you a more sophisticated answer. In the past, the pharmaceutical industry was not able to show the benefit for patients. This is probably related to the tradition of the pharmaceutical industry in Germany, where they have very high research ethics. The argument used by the German pharmaceutical industry was: 'We are doing research. We spend a lot on research and we have good researchers and good professionals.' The target of this message was the decision-makers in medical care, who understand research and its outcomes. Currently, however, research and science have a relatively low status in Germany compared to other countries. In addition, the politics are being conducted by others who do not have a research and science background, so they are not impressed by this message. A new terminology has to be developed, one which explains the benefits of the pharmaceutical industry, but with more thought being given to the patient than to the decision-makers and the key players in the medical arena.

The new reference price system: now and in the future

Q: Do you think that there will be any price/volume controls for the products not subject to reference prices in Germany?

A: I think that ultimately the reference price system will cover almost the entire market. There will not be any products left outside the reference price system. That is the discussion currently taking place in Germany.

Q: Following the previous comment, if the reference price system becomes quasi-universal, it needs to be changed, because of the way it is currently defined. New products cannot be included, unless they are a close product within the ATC* code. Do you think a change in the system is needed to cover that?

A: It is a question of definition. You can now group three products under patent together under the same reference price group, if you can argue that they have almost the same medical efficacy. Only unique innovations are outside this. You can also restrict the grouping of products under patent to two products which have the same performance. There are many ways to define the difference(s) between products in order to avoid being grouped together under one reference price. I think that in the future the reference price system will be extended and, where there are some products left out, perhaps the French system will be adopted.

Q: What are the specific criteria regarding the grouping of certain drugs in Germany? Is there one single most important criterion that determines whether a medicine is introduced in a big 'jumbo' cluster?

* ATC = Anatomical Therapeutic Chemical Classification System

A: It is up to the federal commission to decide which medicines are grouped under the same reference price. This decision is (partially) based on health technology assessment studies, i.e. whether there are large benefit differences between different drugs.

Q: So cost-effectiveness studies are crucial in the definition of these groups.

A: They are crucial, and they will play a really dominant role in the future.

Q: Of the features of the reference price system, which are the ones which have attracted most opposition? Which are the ones that are reasonably easy to sell to the industry and to people within the system?

A: I do not know if I am the right person to answer this question, because I do not work for the pharmaceutical industry. If you have a governmental health insurance scheme where they use the market to buy products, they need some kind of reference price for what they buy. The basic idea of the system therefore is very straightforward. It is also straightforward to set a reference price which says: 'We reimburse the patient only that amount of money and, if the price is higher, the patient has to pay the excess out of pocket.' The problems are in the details. If you include numerous and varied drugs in one large group, and then set a reference price for this group, you have an unfair situation where the pharmaceutical industry can end up not investing in R&D.

Physician drug budgets

Q: Will the individual physician budgets that you mentioned be adjusted by physician specialty and by the demographics of the physician's patients? If not, is there a concern about cream-skimming and lack of access for chronically ill patients?

A: Currently the budgets for physicians are specified by the specialty of the physician. So a gynaecologist has a different budget to an internist or a psychiatrist. They are not adjusted by the age structure of the patients. However, if the physician is above his budget then he can claim, by filling out some forms, that he has a very special patient group. There are a lot of chronic diseases which are exempted from this individual drug budget; for instance, HIV patients, CF patients or diabetes patients.

Q: Is there some sort of punishment for overspending and overprescribing physicians?

A: Yes, physicians are fined if they overprescribe. There is a formal process. They are first asked why they have overprescribed; then they fill out the forms. They have an appearance at the medical doctors' association, and then they are fined.

Q: Do you have any data on these fines? It seems to be a very lengthy process.

A: Three per cent of the physicians receive fines annually – but many more have to fill out forms. A very small percentage of physicians pay fines but, as with car drivers, it is enough to encourage them to stick to the speed limits.

Fragmentation of the German healthcare system

Q: I still have this instinctive impression of the German healthcare system as being very fragmented. You talked a little about the consolidation of the insurers providing an opportunity to manage the system. Is Germany going to have more integrated care and develop disease management programmes?

A: Yes, they are trying to integrate healthcare. It has been argued over the last 20 years that the German system is segmented, and there have been a large number of government initiatives to overcome this segmentation. There are two large programmes. One is the managed care programme, which is financed by our redistribution fund. Although difficult to explain, the essence of the programme is that whenever there are a number of sickness funds, those people who are insured can choose the fund. Then, the fund with young healthy males is much better off. There are therefore redistribution programmes among these funds, and part of the money is taken in order to finance the managed care programmes. Second, there is an integrated care programme. One per cent of the remuneration going to hospitals and physicians is deducted and spent on these integrated healthcare programmes. Both programmes have ended up in a big administration. The question is if they really will lead to a more integrated healthcare system, or simply that the suppliers of healthcare will try to get money from the sickness funds.

References

Eberhardt S, Stocklossa C and Graf von der Schulenburg J-M (eds) (2004) *EUROMET 2004: the influence of economic evaluation studies on healthcare decision making, biomedical and health research.* IOS Press, Amsterdam.

Graf von der Schulenburg J-M (ed.) (2000) *The Influence of Economic Evaluation Studies on Healthcare Decision Making, Biomedical and Health Research.* IOS Press, Amsterdam.

Graf von der Schulenburg J-M and Blanke M (eds) (2004) *Rationing of Medical Services in Europe: an empirical study, biomedical and health research.* IOS Press, Amsterdam.

Kulp W, Greiner W, Graf von der Schulenburg J-M (2005) Nutzenbewertung von Arzneimitteln durch das Institute for Quality and Efficiency in Medical Care (IQWiG) an beispiel der statine. *Perfusion.* **18**.

CHAPTER 3

Pricing and reimbursement policies in the UK: current and future trends

Martina Garau and Adrian Towse

This chapter describes the UK regulatory framework in the pharmaceutical sector, highlighting some of the issues around the policy measures introduced in the country and outlining some possible developments.

Overview of the UK pharmaceutical market

The National Health Service (NHS) budget has been increasing by about 10% per annum in nominal terms. Given that general price inflation has been about 2.5%, the real increases in NHS spending have been around 7% to 7.5%. This has been a deliberate injection of increased public funding in order to raise UK levels to the EU average. As a consequence, pharmaceutical spend, which has been growing at less than 10% per annum, has declined slightly as a share of NHS spend over the last five years. In 2005, because of the 7% price cut imposed by the new Pharmaceutical Price Regulation Scheme (PPRS) (discussed in more detail below), pharmaceutical expenditure will fall further as a proportion of total NHS spending.

We now present some evidence comparing medicines' price levels and pharmaceutical consumption in the UK with other countries. The UK government publishes each year a Report to Parliament on the PPRS. These reports include, among other things, an international price comparison of branded pharmaceuticals. The most recent report, published in March 2005, stated that 'UK prices are higher than all other European countries'. This was at the time the Department of Health was introducing a 7% price cut – so you can understand why they wanted to stress that point. Table 3.1 replicates the results found in the 2005 Report to Parliament regarding bilateral comparisons of prices.

TABLE 3.1 Bilateral comparison of ex-manufacturer prices

Country	1999	2000	2001	2002	2003	Five-year average*
France	84	80	81	81	91	84
Germany	97	91	94	95	102	94
Italy	83	79	82	86	90	83
Netherlands	NA	81	84	88	93	85
Spain	67	64	67	75	81	74
UK	100	100	100	100	100	100
US	184	209	217	201	190	210
Austria	83	77	81	86	94	86
Belgium	84	78	81	86	91	83
Finland	85	83	84	88	98	90
Ireland	88	83	88	93	NA	NA

NA, not available.

*Uses 2003 price information but converted to sterling, for this comparison, using the average exchange rate for the period 1999–2003.

Source: Department of Health (2005).

The international price comparisons found in these reports to Parliament compare the prices of all preparations for the top 150 branded medicines in the UK with other countries, depending on the availability of matching preparations elsewhere. The final column of Table 3.1 shows the price indices for 2003 using a five-year average exchange rate – this is effectively the basis of the Department of Health's quote mentioned above. The UK price index, at 100, is higher than the other European countries included in the sample. Looking at the 2003 data in Table 3.1 at current UK exchange rates, prices in the UK are slightly below Germany and around the same level as Finland. The study does not include Sweden and Switzerland, which are two of the higher-priced European countries.

These price comparisons have to be put in the context of relatively lower volumes of pharmaceuticals sales in the UK. Figure 3.1, which combines Intercontinental Medical Statistics (IMS) and Organization for Economic Cooperation and Development (OECD) data, shows pharmaceutical per capita spend in a number of countries. The UK is towards the bottom end. The UK is therefore characterised by relatively high prices and relatively low volumes in the branded market.

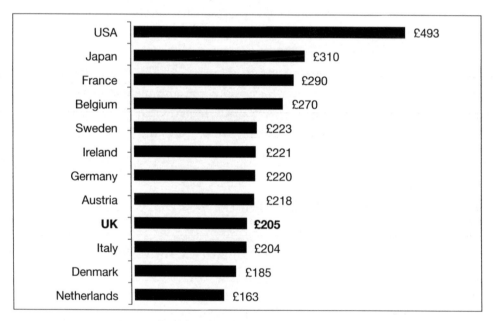

FIGURE 3.1   Pharmaceutical expenditure, per head, 2004. Source: Office of Health Economics (2005).

In the context of branded medicines, it is important to emphasise that prices are not directly controlled at launch in the UK. Companies can fix the price of their new products, provided that:

▸ any subsequent price increase is first approved by the Department of Health

▸ the rate of return limits imposed by the PPRS agreements are not broken.

In addition, companies ought to consider that the price they set at launch may influence the outcome of any cost-effectiveness evaluations of their products conducted by the National Institute for Health and Clinical Excellence (NICE), the Scottish Medicines Consortium (SMC) and the All-Wales Medicines Strategy Group (AWMSG), which issue recommendations on the use of health technologies within their respective parts of the NHS. Price affects a medicine's cost-effectiveness and this, in turn, could influence significantly the outcome of the decision-making processes of NICE, the SMC and the AWMSG.

In essence, NICE (England and Wales), SMC (Scotland) and AWMSG (Wales) have been created to provide recommendations on the most appropriate use of health technologies within the NHS on the basis of clinical and cost-effectiveness evidence. The remits of these institutes are, among others, to appraise the cost-effectiveness of health technologies and to establish whether or not these products provide good value for money for the NHS.

NICE makes decisions on both old and new technologies which are in essence selected by ministers in England and Wales, while the SMC issues guidance on all newly licensed medicines, new indications and formulations. The AWMSG is similar to the SMC as it looks at new products; in particular, it considers high-cost products, defined as products associated with a cost to the NHS exceeding £2000 per patient per year.

Recent changes in P&R regulation
Branded medicines: the PPRS

The PPRS and its predecessors have regulated the UK market since 1955. It is a voluntary agreement between the Association of the British Pharmaceutical Industry (ABPI) and the Department of Health (on behalf of the health ministers of all the countries of the UK) which aims at securing:

▶ safe and effective medicines at a reasonable price

▶ a strong and profitable pharmaceutical industry

▶ an efficient and competitive development and supply of medicines.

It covers all licensed branded prescription medicines sold to the NHS (80% of the NHS medicines bill in terms of value in 2004). The PPRS does not cover unbranded generics or over-the-counter (OTC) products.

According to the current PPRS agreement, which covers the period 2005–2009, firms are allowed to set the price of new products freely, subject to a target rate on return of capital employed (ROCE) of 21%. Around this 21% target there is an upper margin of tolerance of 140% and a lower margin of tolerance of 40%. If a company exceeds 140% of the profit target (i.e. a ROCE above 29.4%), it has to cut its prices or refund the surplus to the Department of Health. On the other hand, if the profit of a company falls below 40% of the 21% target rate (i.e. ROCE below 8.4%), the firm can apply for a price increase that can take this company to 65% of this 21% target. Alternatively, scheme members with little capital in the UK are assessed on a return on sales (ROS) basis, and the target rate of profit is 6% of sales, with equivalent margins of tolerance.

There are certain cost allowances when profits are assessed. For instance, the PPRS allows up to 28% of NHS sales for R&D expenditure. This R&D allowance has three elements:

▶ a flat rate (up to 20% of total NHS sales for assessing profits)

▶ a variable rate for innovation (up to 5%)

▶ a variable rate for paediatrics (1% for each product with a marketing authorisation including a paediatric indication, up to three products a year).

Allowable sales promotion expenses are calculated using a fixed element of £1 million and 4% of NHS sales, plus a small allowance for each molecule. Finally, companies' permitted costs include an allowance for information, up to 4% of NHS sales.

The PPRS not only sets limits on the rate of return that can be earned by individual companies from branded sales to the NHS but also requires them to reduce the price of their branded products at the start of each new scheme. For instance, the latest PPRS agreement imposed an across-the-board price cut of 7% at the start of the new scheme. Nevertheless, the price modulation arrangements allow companies a certain degree of flexibility to decide which products should be sold at a lower price and by how much, as long as the company delivers an overall 7% price reduction. This is also valid for subsequent price changes, where they have to ensure that the overall effect to the NHS is cost neutral.

P&R policies and companies' entry and pricing behaviour

We now want to discuss how these policies have affected the UK market. In Chapter 6, Patricia Danzon discusses the results of a study which essentially looks at the relationship between the degree of price regulation and delays in launch around the world (Danzon *et al.*, 2005). What this study shows is that the UK had the most potential launches and the shortest average launch delays, that is, between when the product was first launched anywhere in the world and when it was launched in the UK. What this suggests is that the freedom of pricing and the speed of entry that the PPRS allows mean that, as a consequence, UK patients get rapid access to products and access to more global products than most European countries.

Looking at the speed of entry and pricing as a consequence, there are two studies that suggest that the speed of second and third entrants coming into a new therapy class in the UK has become more rapid (Reekie, 1996; Towse and Leighton, 1999). What also seems to have been happening is that, whereas in the 1960s, 1970s and to some extent in the 1980s, when a second and third entrant came into a marketplace they were typically priced above the first entrant to try and signal superior quality; the convention in the 1990s and in the current decade is that they are priced at the same level or below the price of the market leaders. There has been a transformation in the way in which companies set entry prices under the PPRS.

We have to put that in context. A series of joint competition studies that were undertaken by the Department of Health and the industry association, the ABPI, in 2002 after the 1999 PPRS negotiations show that the extent of price change within the UK marketplace is relatively limited (DoH and ABPI, 2002). Most price reductions occur as a consequence of the overall price cuts imposed at the start of each of the previous PPRSs: 2.5% in 1993 and 4.5% in 1999.

Essentially, as we might expect, it is partly a one-shot game. Setting the entry price is very important to companies because the opportunity to change that price subsequently is relatively limited. There is some price competition around, but it is limited. There is a difference of emphasis between the industry and the government on the extent to which the PPRS is constraining price competition – with the Department of Health arguing that it is not and the industry arguing that it is.

Generic medicines: the W and M schemes

In June 2005, new arrangements replaced previous systems for generics, introducing categories M and W of the Drug Tariff. Within this new system, the Department of Health will gather volume and value sales data to determine the Drug Tariff price to be reimbursed to pharmacists.* It is important to highlight that companies will now need to submit information on price levels net of discounts. Previously, companies

---

* The interested reader can find more information on the UK generic market in Mestre-Ferrandiz (2006).

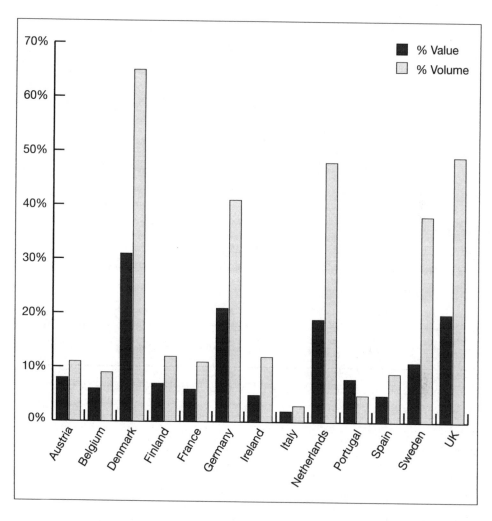

FIGURE 3.2   Generic market shares across Europe, 2004. Source: European Generic Medicines Association (EGA) website (www.egagenerics.com).

did not have to submit information on the level of discounts given to pharmacists. In practice, companies will compete to supply pharmacists with generics below the price set by the Drug Tariff.

The reimbursed prices of generics are determined by the Drug Tariff. Alongside Drug Tariff, the other element influencing the generics prices paid by the NHS is the discount claw-back of pharmacists' margins. As pharmacists and dispensing doctors are reimbursed at the fixed Drug Tariff price but buy generic products at a discounted price (around 15% on average below the list price), they have an incentive to try and obtain the largest discounts possible and to dispense the product that provides them with the highest profit margin.

In this context, the main challenges for the Department of Health in getting value for money in the generics segment in the UK have been transaction prices being much lower than list prices and the presence of some price volatility. There were large increases in the prices of some generics in 1999. As a result of these price increases, a Maximum Price Scheme was introduced in 2000 as a temporary measure for all generic products. In essence, the Maximum Price Scheme constrained generic prices to their pre-shock, that is, 1998/1999 levels. As a result of the subsequent review of the generics market carried out by the Department of Health, generic companies now have to submit data on discounts in exchange for more pricing freedom as a result of the new M and W categories.

Figure 3.2 shows the market share of generics, both in terms of volume and value, across a number of European countries in 2004. From Figure 3.2 we can see that, roughly speaking, Europe is divided in half. The UK, Sweden, Netherlands, Germany and Denmark have very strong generics markets: strong in terms of volume but also because those generics are supplied at relatively low prices compared to branded products. In the UK, for instance, generics account for nearly 50% in volume terms, but around 20% in value terms. The UK is one of the few countries in Europe that has a very competitive generics market. One can see that France is towards the bottom end of the European countries in terms of the value of the generics market, at well under 10%.

Prescribers and dispensers

The current regulatory framework in the UK enables doctors to prescribe medicines using their international non-proprietary names (INN). Indeed, generic prescribing is very common in the UK, with 80% of NHS prescriptions written generically. However, pharmacists are not allowed to dispense a medicine other than that prescribed if not authorised by the doctor, that is, generic substitution by pharmacists is not allowed.

Prescribing choices are also influenced by:

▶ a negative list, which includes drugs that should not be prescribed by doctors on behalf of the NHS

▶ a restricted use list, which includes drugs that should only be prescribed if certain conditions are met; an example of a drug included in this list is Viagra.

It should be noted that these two lists do not have as significant an impact on the UK market as they do in many other countries, such as Spain.

Other measures influencing prescription behaviour include the following.

▶ GP prescribing budgets. Policy reforms introduced in the NHS in 1990 allocated purchasing power and budgets to primary care physicians – so-called fundholding GPs – to buy hospital services and pharmaceuticals. GP fundholding was brought to an end in 1999 by the new Labour government. But now practice-based commissioning is being introduced and is to be implemented by the end of 2006. As part of this the Department of Health allocates an annual budget to each primary care trust (PCT) covering a given geographical area. Then each PCT allocates indicative budgets to individual practices, which will be responsible for managing the demands of healthcare services for the local populations, including medicines, within these budgets.

▶ Prescribing incentive schemes, which allow PCTs and primary care organisations (PCOs) to work directly with general practices and primary care professionals to improve service delivery.

▶ Information and education campaigns.

▶ Clinical practice guidelines issued by NICE and the Scottish Intercollegiate Guidelines Network (SIGN), and National Service Frameworks (NSFs), which set national standards for a defined service or care group.

The last two are non-financial measures which aim, inter alia, at promoting good prescribing practice.

NICE and the use of cost-effectiveness analysis

NICE (in England and Wales) is applying cost-effectiveness criteria by first looking at the clinical evidence and other related evidence on effects and costs and then saying, 'Here's our estimate of effects; here's our estimate of costs. Does it represent value for money for the NHS?' Many of you will be aware of the debate as to whether NICE has a threshold and exactly what it is. Towse *et al.* (2002) show some evidence on this matter. Initially, Michael Rawlins, Chair of NICE, made a comment that, as an observation, there seemed to be a cut-off point of around £30 000 per QALY. Products below this level were likely to get through whilst products above it were much less likely to get through.

The new guide NICE has published (NICE, 2004) for manufacturers and other institutions interested in making submissions to NICE when technologies are appraised, explicitly indicates a threshold varying between £20 000 and £30 000: below £20 000 there is a high chance of acceptance; above £30 000 there is a low chance of acceptance. Recent studies have attempted, using econometric methods, to analyse the extent to which cost-effectiveness appears to be influencing decisions (Devlin and Parkin, 2004; Dakin *et al.*, 2006).

Figure 3.3 shows a graph extracted from Rawlins and Culyer (2004) that illustrates the relationship between the probability of a technology being rejected on the ground of cost-effectiveness and its incremental cost-effectiveness ratio.

We have a situation in which there is no single cut-off point, but the probability of rejection on the grounds of cost-effectiveness increases as the cost per QALY increases. NICE is signalling very clearly – both from its past behaviour and from the outline guidance given to manufacturers – that below £20 000 there is a high chance of acceptance, and that above £30 000 there is a low chance of acceptance. However, it does not mean that a technology will always be accepted if its cost-effectiveness ratio is below £20 000 per QALY, and it does not mean that it will not be accepted if it is above £30 000 per QALY.

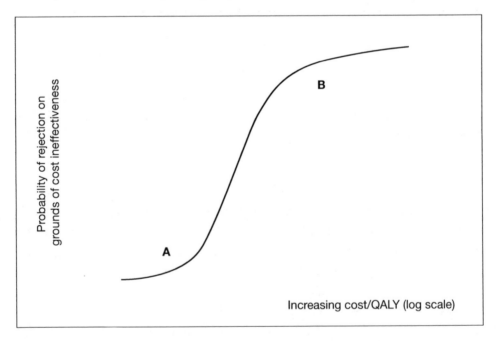

FIGURE 3.3   Relation between likelihood of a technology being considered as cost ineffective plotted against the log of the incremental cost-effectiveness ratio. Source: Rawlins and Culyer (2004).

As far as NICE is concerned the UK environment is characterised by a significant degree of transparency in terms of what the basis will be on which NICE will make positive or negative recommendations as to whether new products should be used by the NHS. We have a complement to the PPRS profit control scheme that permits freedom of pricing at launch, because that freedom is constrained by an increasingly active value-for-money agency saying, 'Given this price, does the technology represent value for money for the NHS?'

NICE and the take-up of medicines

Sheldon and colleagues have carried out some work for NICE looking at the take-up of products recommended by NICE. The results have been published in the *British Medical Journal* (Sheldon *et al.*, 2004) and Figures 3.4 and 3.5 below are extracted from it.

Figure 3.4 shows the example of orlistat, an anti-obesity product. You can see the jump in uptake when the NICE guidance came out in March 2001.

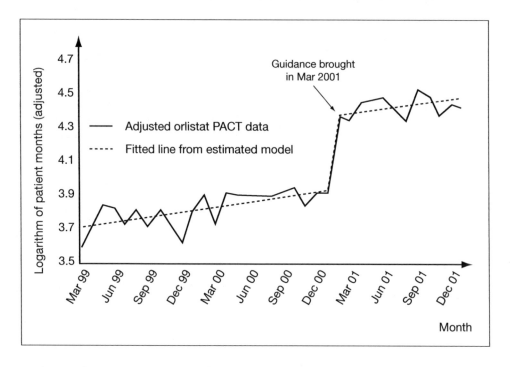

FIGURE 3.4   Use of orlistat in the community. Source: Sheldon *et al.* (2004).

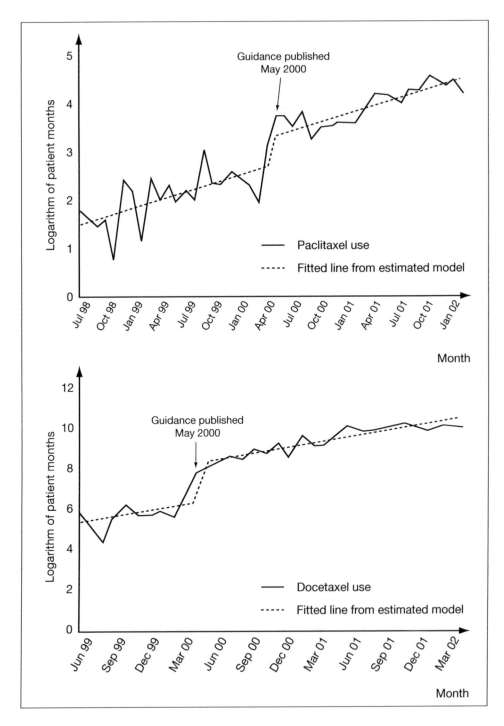

FIGURE 3.5 Hospital use of paclitaxel (top) and docetaxel (bottom). Source: Sheldon *et al.* (2004).

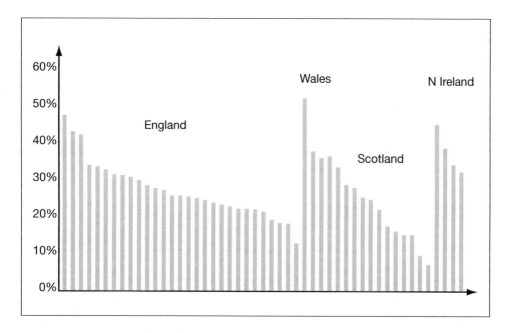

FIGURE 3.6   Obesity drug – patient penetration, July–March 2004. Source: Roche
(2004).

Figure 3.5 displays the situation with two taxanes; again, there is an increase in
take-up when the NICE decisions come out (May 2000).

There are other examples in the paper by Sheldon *et al.* (2004), however, where
the implementation of NICE decisions has not taken place and therefore has not
been effective.

Figure 3.6 show an analysis of a Roche product that Roche has shared with NICE,
which illustrates the degree of patient penetration. It relates to different areas of,
respectively, England, Wales, Scotland and Northern Ireland. Figure 3.6 shows a
huge differentiation in the extent of take-up and implementation of NICE decisions
across different parts of the UK. It is giving a rough indication of the dispersal of use.
We have a situation in which the implementation of NICE guidance by the NHS is
varied. For some products it works well but, even in those products where it works
well, there is a large divergence in uptake from place to place. In other products, it
does not work well at all.

We seem to have a situation where there is a missing link. We have a profit
control; we have value for money tests for new products, linked to freedom of
pricing; but we do not seem to have a mechanism which is currently working

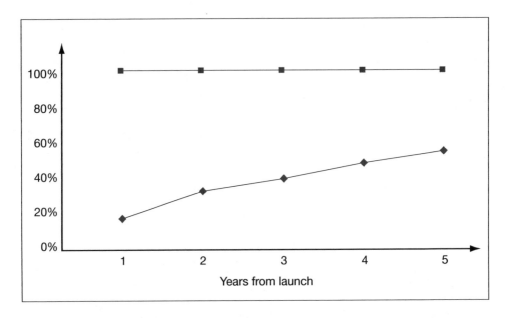

FIGURE 3.7   UK update (◆) of new medicines launched in the UK since 1998 compared to average for other Pharmaceutical Industry Competitive Task Force (PICTF) countries (■). Source: PICTF (2005), Indicator 16.

properly whereby those products that NICE says represent value for money are necessarily being taken up by the NHS.

Figure 3.7 shows the results of work done by the industry, the Department of Health and other government departments: a benchmarking exercise that came out of the Pharmaceutical Industry Competitive Task Force (PICTF), which was commissioned by the Prime Minister in 2000. This analysis has been updated every year since then. Figure 3.7 shows how the uptake in the UK of new medicines launched since 1998 compares to a number of countries.

From the latest analysis, and looking at the comparator countries in terms of take-up of new medicines launched since 1998, the UK is under 40% of the level of other countries three years after launch. Thus, take-up of new medicines is an issue in the UK shared by government and industry alike.

Target of national health policy

Table 3.2 summarises the mechanisms the UK government relies on to control the pharmaceutical market.

TABLE 3.2 Target of national health policy

Supply-side			Demand-side		
Price		**Profit control**	**Volume control**	**Prescribers/ dispensers**	**Patients**
Direct	**Indirect**				
PPRS price cut of branded medicines	NICE/SMC recommendations based on economic evaluation	PPRS rate of return	Negative list	GP budgets and prescribing incentive schemes NICE/SMC guidance on use Clinical practice guidance	Fixed prescription charge

PPRS, Pharmaceutical Price Regulation Scheme; NICE/SMC, National Institute for Clinical Excellence/Scottish Medicines Consortium.

On the supply side we have the PPRS, which has a significant direct impact on price and the rate of return; there is then the indirect effect of the NICE decision-making process, which is based on cost-effectiveness evaluations; and then there is the negative list, which has only a minor impact.

On the demand side we have the sizeable impact of GP budgets and prescribing incentive schemes and, indirectly, NICE and SMC recommendations, which influence prescribing behaviour, as well as clinical practice guidance. The fixed prescription charge does not play a significant role, as almost 85% of the prescribed items are dispensed free of charge to the 50% of the population who are exempt from paying prescription charges.

National P&R policies in the future

Before discussing what the future could hold for the UK's pharmaceutical market, we need to stress that the regulatory framework, as a consequence of the PPRS which is fixed for a five-year period, is a stable environment which seems to have successfully promoted long-term investment. The UK pharmaceutical industry has under 4% of the global pharmaceutical market but around 10% of global R&D. Essentially, therefore, the UK is getting nearly three times its market share in terms of R&D. Obviously, the science base and other characteristics of the UK environment are key factors driving this result, but industry and government see the PPRS also as an important factor.

Let us focus now on the future. Considering the generics sector first, we have had a new regimen since mid-2005. It is linked to the new pharmacy contracting arrangements. One can expect these new arrangements to remain relatively stable for the next few years.

In terms of the PPRS, we also have a new scheme – which we might have expected would mean that we had a relatively stable environment. However, in 2004, the Office of Fair Trading (OFT) undertook an overview of government procurement. It identified eight or nine sectors where there was potential concern as to whether the supply conditions in those sectors were sufficiently good to ensure that government was getting value for money. One of the sectors was pharmaceuticals. The OFT has been carrying out investigations into a number of those sectors and announced in September 2005 that it was going to look at pharmaceuticals as part of that rolling programme. As a consequence it is carrying out a market review, which is essentially looking at whether the PPRS is meeting its objectives – in terms of value for money for the NHS, competition in the supply of medicines, rewards to research and a strong and profitable industry. The issues will be around whether the government is getting value for money through the PPRS in terms of achieving those objectives, and the extent to which the market is as competitive as it could be.

There are obviously varying types of recommendations that the OFT could make. In terms of what might happen to the PPRS, therefore, we have a new scheme but there is a degree of uncertainty as to whether that scheme will run its full five-year term without amendment.

The third topic to discuss is NICE. There are continuing issues regarding the speed with which NICE makes decisions and whether those decisions are then taken up. This has led to NICE proposing a new technology appraisal mechanism: a rapid (single technology) appraisal, which will enable it to issue faster guidance on new treatments or on existing drugs with new indications.

We are also seeing the growing importance of clinical practice guidelines, which are part of the NICE remit. NICE is increasingly seeking to slot the individual product technology appraisals into its clinical practice guidelines; that is, not just 'Should Product X be used – yes or no?' but 'What should be the process of caring for the patient, and where does Product X fit into that?' We are seeing quite a significant shift in emphasis in NICE, with potentially a greater role for economic evaluation within the UK, as part of the development by NICE, and use by the NHS, of clinical practice guidelines.

Again, there are the issues of implementation. We have seen some of the issues with respect to the implementation of technology appraisals. There are many more issues of implementation with respect to clinical practice guidelines. Although the work is being done nationally, the extent to which that will influence patterns of clinical behaviour as yet remains unknown.

Finally in relation to NICE we seem to be seeing an increasingly explicit threshold and a greater transparency of the criteria that are being used.

In the NHS, we will see more pressure on budgets in the future. The next government three-year spending review will take place in 2006/07, governing NHS spending from 2007 onwards. NHS spending growth has been running at 10% in nominal terms; that is, 7.5% real. The expectation is that growth rates may well be halved from 2008 onwards. NHS spending would then be rising by 5% per year, equal to about 2.5% real, which will have a dramatic effect on the cost pressures the NHS faces, and on the ability and willingness of the NHS to prescribe medicines.

That is linked to another attempt by the Department of Health to revisit demand-side management. Primarily, the Department is concerned with managing the commissioning of care from hospitals and trying to give GPs greater control over that, through reforms to PCTs and the introduction of practice-based commissioning. This will mean that GP prescribing budgets will be under much more scrutiny within primary care; GPs will face direct incentives; and GP-led commissioners will be able to shift money into and out of prescribing, into and out of hospital care.

What we may well see are pressures on prescribing that we have not seen in the UK for the last four years – because of the deliberately rapid growth in NHS spending – both in terms of pressure on budgets and also in terms of new management arrangements in primary care.

Discussion

The claw-back system and how it has evolved in the new pharmacy contract

Q: You indicated that a claw-back system applies to generics. My understanding is that this system is implemented for all drugs, including branded drugs. Is that correct?

Q: My second question is related to the new pharmacy contract. Have the claw-back system and margins changed in the latest contract?

A: The claw-back mechanism does not cover only generics; it covers all pharmacy purchases. There is therefore a continuing incentive for wholesalers to compete by offering discounts to pharmacists, and for pharmacists to be shop-ping around in terms of which wholesaler they use and, obviously, in terms of generics and parallel trade, which suppliers they use.

Regarding your second question, my understanding is that a broad sum of money was agreed for the total of all pharmacy services and, within that, there were certain changes to what pharmacists would be rewarded for. One of the big changes goes back to our presentation of the new generics scheme, where the Department of Health is trying to introduce a new pricing mechanism that is better at tracking underlying transaction prices. There should be smaller discounts within the system. As a consequence, therefore, that part of pharmacy remuneration arising from discounts inevitably would be expected to come down, and other parts to increase.

Ex-manufacturer prices versus public prices

Q: I have a comment on the price comparison in Europe. I fully agree that ex-factory prices in the UK are the highest in Europe. However, if you consider public prices, namely prices including taxation and distribution margins, the situation changes significantly. First of all, unlike other continental countries, VAT is not added to drugs prices in the UK. Second, the distribution margins are much lower in the UK compared to other nations, thanks to its very effective and efficient claw-back system. To summarise, the UK high ex-manufacturer prices are mitigated, if not compensated, by distribution margins, which is a critical issue still pending in most continental countries.

A: If you look at IMS public prices as opposed to IMS ex-manufacturer, then you do get a different distribution of prices, and the UK distribution system is one of the most efficient in Europe.

The slow uptake of new medicines and the extent to which it is due to a NICE dysfunction

Q: Could you comment on the phenomenon of 'NICE blight'? I am reminded of this by your reference to the slow rate of uptake of new medicines in the UK compared with other economies. A supplementary question would be this. I can understand why doctors may be reluctant to prescribe a medicine or a group of medicines if it is known that NICE is undertaking a review – because they do not know what the outcome will be – but is there any evidence that they are reluctant to prescribe new drugs per se, because they simply do not know whether or not NICE will want to examine that group of drugs? How far do you connect 'NICE blight' with the continued reluctance of the UK market to take up new medicines?

A: There is a situation in which prescribers either think that something has been referred to NICE or are expecting something to be referred to NICE – or indeed they think that something should be referred to NICE. In this context, it is important to understand if this leads to a period where there is very little prescribing, or indeed where there are active attempts to stop prescribing until NICE has made a decision.

The evidence suggests that this has been happening but it is not universal. The picture varies by product.

Clearly, this is one of the things which has led to pressure from government and from industry to get NICE to reform the speed with which it reviews products. Part of the pressure from the Department of Health and from industry for changes in NICE processes, therefore, has been to try to tackle that problem of delay, or the lack of clarity as to what people should do in the intervening period.

Does that explain the low prescribing rates and low take-up of new products? The reality is that low uptake predates the introduction of NICE. Indeed, one of the precipitating reasons for NICE was that the Department of Health wanted to have a more consistent take-up of new medicines that represented good value for money for the NHS. What the implementation slides show is that it is still a mixed picture. Even where we have a positive NICE recommendation, we are still meeting some resistance – whether that is from prescribing clinicians, or budgetary concerns on the part of the PCTs and the hospitals. Again, reasons probably vary from product to product.

So there is something called 'NICE blight', and that is one of the reasons for the proposed changes in NICE processes. Is that the reason for low UK prescribing? No. NICE is one of the mechanisms that are meant to speed it up. What we are seeing is that it is having some success in speeding it up, but there is still some way to go.

NICE budget cuts
Q: I want to raise a point about these rumoured, and published, budget cuts in the NICE process. A key aspect of the evidence model was that they had independent HTA review. I am interested to hear your insights as to whether,

with less money being available, this changes the onus more towards the industry presenting the evidence. How does that relate to the single drug review?

A: I do find it bizarre that the Department of Health is putting a lot of pressure on the NICE budget in real terms. Given the importance of having good HTA and an understanding of whether technologies represent value for money, given the potential for achieving health gains or savings depending on whether or not they are cost-effective, it would seem to me that, strategically, one would want to be spending more rather than less.

That is only part of the reason for the 'single technology appraisal' proposals. Part of the issue is that, if you go for a more rapid review, you have to take some work out of the process. Part of it, therefore, is trying to think through how to have a more rapid HTA process. One route is to put more emphasis on the industry presentation of evidence – as is the case with the SMC process. My understanding – and clearly NICE is still developing these proposals – is that there will be an opportunity to revisit the appraisal at a later date, if there are issues of substance that require more analysis, or indeed more evidence. One needs to separate the budget element from what you have to do in order to get through the process more quickly – although clearly they are partly related.

The role of independent HTA review in the NICE appraisal process
Q: Is there any sense that the industry will lose out by having less rigorous treatment from independent HTA agencies?

A: Is a process that is more manufacturer-driven a better or a worse one? We have different models around the world and it is difficult to separate them from their institutional setting. It seems to me that the manufacturer submission should play a crucial role. Likewise, some independent review of the quality of that submission, and of other data, if available, supporting the same or different result, is also very important.

References

Dakin HA, Devlin NJ and Odeyemi IAO (2006) 'Yes', 'No' or 'YES, but'? Multinomial modelling of NICE decision-making. *Health Policy.* **77**(3): 352–67.

Danzon P, Wang R and Wang L (2005) The impact of price regulation on the launch delay of new drugs. *Health Economics.* **14**: 269–92.

Department of Health and ABPI (2002) *Study into the Extent of Competition in the Supply of Branded Medicines to the NHS.* Department of Health, London.

Department of Health (2005) *Pharmaceutical Price Regulation Scheme. Eighth Report to Parliament.* Department of Health, London.

Devlin N and Parkin D (2004) Does NICE have a cost-effectiveness threshold and what other factors influence its decisions? A binary choice analysis. *Health Economics.* **13**: 437–52.

Mestre-Ferrandiz J (2006) *The Faces of Regulation: profit and price regulation of the UK pharmaceutical industry after the 1998 Competition Act.* Office of Health Economics, London.

National Institute for Clinical Excellence (2004) *Guide to the Methods of Technology Appraisal.* NICE, London.

Office of Health Economics (2005) *OHE Compendium of Health Statistics.* Office of Health Economics, London.

Pharmaceutical Industry Competitiveness Task Force (2005) *Competitiveness and Performance Indicators, 2005.* PICTF, Department of Health, London.

Rawlins MD and Culyer AJ (2004) National Institute for Clinical Excellence and its value judgements. *BMJ.* **329**: 224–27.

Reekie WE (1996) *Medicine Prices and Innovations. An International Survey.* IEA Health and Welfare Unit, London.

Roche (2004) Presentation: Audit into the implementation of NICE guidance for Roche drugs. Available from: www.nice.org.uk/page.aspx?o=203728 (accessed November 2005).

Sheldon TA, Cullum N, Dawson D, Lankshear A, Lowson K, Watt I *et al.* (2004) What's the evidence that NICE guidance has been implemented? Results from a national evaluation using time series analysis, audit of patients' notes and interviews. *BMJ.* **329**: 999–1007.

Towse A, Pritchard C and Devlin N (2002) *Cost-effectiveness Thresholds. Economic and Ethical Issues.* The King's Fund and Office of Health Economics, London.

Towse A and Leighton T (1999) The changing nature of NICE pricing of second and subsequent entrants. In: Sussex J and Marchant N (1999) *Risk and Return in the Pharmaceutical Industry.* Office of Health Economics, London.

CHAPTER 4

Pricing and reimbursement policies in Italy: current and future trends

Livio Garattini

This chapter describes the Italian pricing and reimbursement system, which is complex because it is constantly changing. It is probably the market in Europe with the most changes, although things seem to be changing constantly everywhere.

Let us begin by describing some general features of the Italian healthcare and the pricing and reimbursement systems. However, the core of this chapter will be on pharmaceutical policy, with the aim of:

▶ stressing the element of novelty introduced in the Italian system, and in particular, the new agency recently created

▶ discussing the main policy laws

▶ describing the generics market, which has now been separated from general pharmaceutical policy.

The chapter concludes by offering some thoughts on possible future scenarios for pricing and reimbursement regulation in Italy.

Overview of the healthcare system in Italy

The Italian National Health Service (NHS) is a three-tier system. This means that the system is modelled in a similar way to that in the UK – although the management is very different. At the top tier the Italian Department of Health is responsible for the planning and allocation of financial resources among regions as well as designing pharmaceutical policy. The second tier involves the regional health authorities (RHAs), which are governed by elected politicians, and whose activities are similar to the English Department of Health but at regional level. Here the difference with the English system is that there are many regional politicians governing the regional health authorities. At the next level, we have the local health authorities (LHAs) and hospital trusts, which are the local tier for providing healthcare services. Both the LHAs and the hospital trusts depend heavily on the regional health authorities because all general managers are appointed by the regional authorities.

In the last decade there have been two major trends in Italy: increased regional autonomy and the introduction of managerial skills at the local level. The first trend is obviously not health-specific. There has been a great deal of discussion about devolution, or federalism; the actual term used usually depends on the political party in question. Significantly, this increased regional autonomy giving regions more financial independence has been recognised through a change to the Constitution. As the healthcare budget represents the largest share of the regional budget, around 80% to 90%, healthcare financing is a significant part of this new autonomy or independence.

In theory, regions are now allowed to collect local taxation and to finance extra healthcare services. RHAs are therefore financially accountable for all of their expenses and particularly for any possible deficit incurred, including pharmaceuticals expenditure. This is a major issue of political debate.

The problem with this devolution is the deficit and, in particular, how it is to be accounted for. First, it is important to define what the deficit is. This is a difficult task because there are many ways in which it can be quantified. Second, the problem is who will pay the deficit. The southern and the central RHAs are all in deficit, and these regions are the poorest in Italy.

The second trend has been to introduce managerial skills at the local level, as happened in the UK in the 1980s with the introduction of general managers. LHAs have been led by general managers appointed by the regional health authorities – making managers dependent on RHAs – with renewable rolling contracts, usually of five years. However, managers can easily be dismissed after elections, subject to the changes in the political party governing the region. One of the objectives of increasing management is to effectively introduce a local budgetary approach, including the costs that are associated with the proportion for pharmaceuticals spend. In principle, this objective should be fulfilled, although we can probably say that this approach is yet to be fully implemented.

So far we have described the current context within Italy's NHS. It is difficult to make predictions about the future because there will be differences between regions, depending on their particular strengths. This will make monitoring the situation more complex.

Overview of the Italian pharmaceutical market

Between 2004 and 2005 the total consumption of pharmaceuticals increased by 2.7%, with a rise of 3.7% for reimbursable medicines and a rise of 1% for non-reimbursable medicines. Looking at the long term (*see* Figure 4.1), we can see total pharmaceutical expenditure fluctuating in both the public and private sectors, mainly due to the introduction of a series of measures aimed at reducing the public healthcare spend.

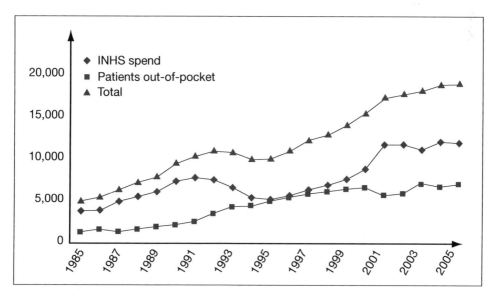

FIGURE 4.1   Long-term trend for the expenditure on pharmaceuticals dispensed by pharmacies in Italy (€, million). Source: CERGAS (2006).

Putting this in an international context (*see* Figure 4.2), it is possible to see that Italy has had one of the lowest average rates of growth of public expenditure per

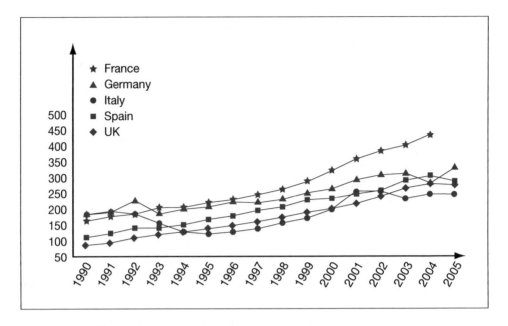

FIGURE 4.2   Public expenditure on pharmaceuticals, per head ($Purchasing Power Parity (PPP)). Source: CERGAS (2006).

capita for pharmaceuticals. This is the result of a combination of measures aimed at reducing the public spend on pharmaceuticals that took place during the first half of the 1990s and in the period after 2001, and of measures that have increased public expenditure in the period between 1996 and 2001.

Current trends in national P&R regulation

Turning to pharmaceutical policy, the real element of novelty in Italy's latest reforms was the setting up of a new national drug agency, *Agenzia Italiana del Farmaco* (AIFA). AIFA is headed by the Ministry of Health and controlled by the Ministry of Economy and regional authorities. The regions and the Ministry of Health find that AIFA has been a good solution to the previous struggle between the national and regional tiers. AIFA allows the regions to play a role in pharmaceutical policy, whereas before the system was managed solely by the Department of Health.

AIFA includes the following areas of activity:

▶ approval and pharmacovigilance

▶ manufacturing control

▶ information and research

▶ pricing, reimbursement and market analysis

▶ assessment of the European procedures.

In principle, AIFA is responsible for all the tasks that a national agency is expected to manage for pharmaceuticals.

Within the Italian pricing and reimbursement system, all new P&R applications are to be submitted to AIFA. Although the name of the agency in charge of such applications has changed, the system remains as it was before, that is, the non-separation between the reimbursement and pricing decisions remains. Although there are now two committees, the Technical Scientific Committee (CTS) and the Pricing and Reimbursement Committee (CPR), they work together within the same organisation.

The new CTS has replaced the *Commissione Unica del Farmaco* (CUF), the former government drug committee. The task of the CTS is to examine dossiers and provide the CPR with an assessment of the efficacy of new drugs. The CPR itself has two main tasks. First, it sets the price of new medicines, and second, it chooses the new medicine's reimbursement class. There are three possible reimbursement classes in Italy:

▶ Class A: fully reimbursed medicines.

▶ Class C: non-reimbursed medicines.

▶ Class H: fully reimbursed hospital-only drugs (although pharmaceutical companies claim that this is not necessarily true).

In practical terms, the more important committee is the CTS, given that its assessments greatly affect the activities and decisions taken by the CPR.

Recent changes in P&R regulation

So far we have illustrated the basic reforms. After the scandal of the bribes which took place in the early 1990s, Italy adopted in 1993 the so-called 'non-price system'. Under this system, officially termed the Average European Price (AEP) system, the price of each medicine was set relative to an average European price. Initially, this average was based on four countries (France, Germany, Spain and the UK) and on exchange rates calculated at purchasing power parities (PPPs). Later it was extended to all European Union (EU) countries. Under this system, during the 1990s, prices that were higher than the resulting AEP had to decrease to the AEP level, whereas prices lower than the AEP were to increase gradually.

Currently, the AEP is no longer used. Given the new (2004) Member States, use of the AEP system could pose serious problems. However, the method is still included in the law and is thus officially in place, but it has not been renewed or updated.

Since 1997, the only real price scheme in place in Italy is the so-called 'contractual model'. Prices of all the new drugs approved through the European centralised procedure, and since 1998 also through the mutual recognition system, have to be negotiated with the national authority – currently AIFA.

There was also an attempt, in 2002, to introduce a sort of 'Level II reference pricing', where different active principals, with overlapping effects in terms of efficacy, were put together into a single reference price group. However, this remained simply an attempt; it was never fully rolled out. It led to the recalculation of prices based on annual turnovers and daily defined doses (DDDs) for those medicines that were going to be subject to this new reference price system. The objective was to set the same price for all products included in the same therapeutic class. It should be pointed out that this reference price system was never intended to include off-patent medicines nor patients' co-payments.

Some initiatives have taken place in order to try and foster R&D in the Italian pharmaceutical market. In 2001, it was decided that innovative drugs would receive a price premium. This policy stated that 'the total budget available should have been shared among manufacturers of new innovative drugs who invest in R&D in Italy'. However, this has not happened in practice so far. In addition, not only was this system never applied, but the total budget for this premium pricing scheme was just 0.1% of total pharmaceutical expenditure – a negligible amount of money.

Expenditure ceilings and price cuts

Let us now turn to what has probably been the most important activity in the Italian pharmaceutical market: a continuous attempt to try to cut prices and to cap expenditure. Starting with budget ceilings, the first attempt at introducing payback mechanisms when actual expenditure exceeds the budget was made in 1997. In principle, 40% of the budget overrun should have been covered by the Italian NHS while the pharmaceutical, wholesale and retail industries were supposed to cover the remaining 60%. But in the event industry, wholesale and retail, did not pay its share.

In 2001 the payback mechanism was changed once again to try to make it more effective, which should not have been a difficult task given the failure of the previous system. Public pharmaceutical expenditure was limited to a share of a maximum of 13% of total regional NHS expenditure. The idea behind this new scheme was to try to make the regional authorities as accountable as possible with regard to their deficit. Nevertheless, the regional expenditure ceiling was changed and moved to a broader budget in 2003. With the new target, overall pharmaceutical expenditure, including both community and hospital expenses, is limited to a maximum of 16% of regional healthcare expenditure.

There have also been several price cuts over the years, starting with a 7% discount for all Class A products and Class H products in 2004. The strongest measure to date was a payback of 6.8% on ex-factory prices on all Class A products, equivalent to a 4.2% reduction in public prices, in 2005. Neither the wholesale nor the retail segment of the market was asked to pay back, only manufacturers. The industry complained and, in this case, they were right. The public price includes distribution margins, and the distribution channel did not have to pay anything back at all. It should be noted that pharmacists usually represent an important lobby, not just in Italy but in all European parliaments.

Prescribers and dispensers

The reforms in Italy allowed local health authorities to introduce expenditure targets and saving incentives to GPs. To date, there is still little evidence that such measures have been successfully applied. Federalism will probably enhance some local activity but at the same time will not ensure any kind of national standard. We are therefore still waiting for some national standards. So far, we are controlling prices in Italy but we still have problems in controlling volumes, as in most European countries, including France and Germany.

Similarly, to date any change in pharmacists' margins has been very modest. In 1997 the retail margin, which up until then was proportional to the retail price, was discounted in favour of the NHS according to defined classes of prices, to achieve a regressive effect. However, the regressive effect was very low. By 2005, the discounts ranged from 3.75% for prices below €25.84 to 19% for products with a price higher than €154.94.

From 2001, regions were allowed to use the so-called 'direct distribution' channel for a limited list of drugs. The aim was to reduce pharmaceutical expenditure by cutting down dispensing prices as a result of using public procurement mechanisms. However, what happened in practice was not what was expected. The pharmacists' lobby was effective in mitigating this very radical change, which would have penalised them quite heavily. There are local health authorities that dispense drugs directly through their facilities, in particular hospitals, bypassing intermediate and retail distribution. However, this form of distribution is rare nowadays as wholesalers and pharmacists negotiate the dispensing of LHA-purchased drugs at much lower margins in order to limit their losses. Pharmacists do not buy the medicines, but rather act as distributors. This system thus gives rise to a double-parallel distribution system and is very difficult to detect because it changes from one region to another. Nevertheless, this 'direct distribution' channel has not been too successful in controlling pharmaceutical expenditure because, eventually, the distribution channel can keep most of the margin, which is why it was stated previously that changes in the distribution sector are not very significant.

The generics market

As illustrated in Chapter 3, the market share of generics in Italy is one of the lowest in Europe. However, it should be highlighted when comparing generic market shares between countries that the definition of 'generics' varies from country to country. Some of the issues regarding generics discussed in this chapter appear in Garattini and Ghislandi (2006). In Italy we have not only generics, but also the so-called 'copies'. These are products which existed before the launch of generics because of insufficient patent laws before the late 1970s. Broadly speaking, these 'copy' products were the result of Italian companies producing (sometimes without permission from the originator company) very similar branded products, because patent laws at the time only applied to process and not product. Partly as a result of weak patent laws, Italy (together with Spain) has experienced more co-marketing strategies for pharmaceuticals. Consequently, there are more copies in the Italian market relative to other markets with stronger patent laws, both as a result of licensed copies and 'old' (i.e. not licensed by the originator company) copies. This can be misleading for international observers, because it is difficult to understand what we mean by 'generics' in Italy.

It was not until 2000 that Italy officially acknowledged the introduction of generics. Level I reference pricing was introduced for off-patent products containing the same active principle. The reference price was set as an average weighted (by volume) price of all drugs included in the same group. However, this system was quickly abandoned because it produced only a very slight decrease in prices. Then a more radical and drastic way of setting the reimbursed price for off-patent drugs was introduced: the cheapest price of the equivalent products in the regional market, that is, the lowest price of the available products. This injected a lot of competitive pricing amongst generics manufacturers. (It is important to emphasise that the reference price in Italy is applied to the same pack size of equivalent products rather than to the same active ingredient.)

Setting the reference price for generics based on the cheapest product was successful in containing pharmaceutical expenditure for high-priced products by cutting down reimbursement prices. Below are three examples showing the price variation for three active ingredients that were subject to this new method of setting the reimbursed price for off-patent medicines. In all three cases, prices fell very dramatically. The first example, shown in Figure 4.3, is ticlopidine.

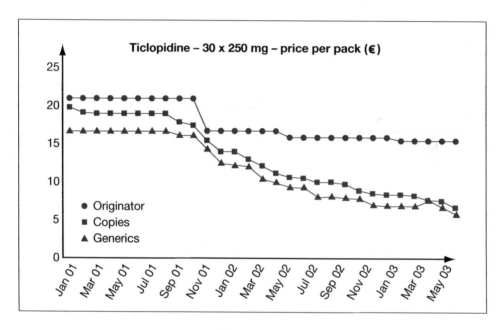

FIGURE 4.3   Price variations for ticlopidine. Source: IMS data.

The original manufacturer was reluctant to decrease the price after cheaper copies and generics were first introduced. It is, however, possible that the Italian affiliate wanted to cut the price, but international headquarters could have other concerns and was thus responsible for this reluctance in cutting the price. I have tried in this example to make a distinction between copies and generics, but it is one where the price for the most-sold pack of ticlopidine (30 x 250 mg) was ultimately decreased dramatically. As illustrated in Figure 4.3, the price of ticlopidine's copies and generics decreased significantly after November 2001, when the reimbursed price was set according to the cheapest products of the group.

Figure 4.4 illustrates the price variation for nimesulide, a very important non-steroidal anti-inflammatory drug (NSAID) in Italy and Spain, although less important in other countries, such as the UK. As illustrated in Figure 4.4 the originator in this case also eventually followed the strategy of cutting prices, because this medicine was important for the company's portfolio strategy.

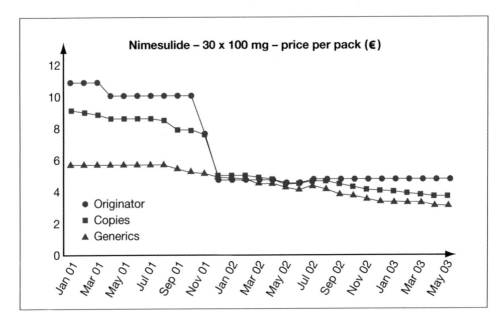

FIGURE 4.4   Price variations for nimesulide. Source: IMS data.

All the price decreases for the active ingredient nimesulide were led by generics manufacturers; copies and originators were only followers of the strategy.

The trend of price for ranitidine, shown in Figure 4.5, differs from the previous two examples for marketing reasons. Here the peculiarity of the ranitidine market in Italy is that the co-marketer of this product used to sell much more than the originator that gave the licence to its Italian partner, so price strategies were affected by this once the patent expired.

Whilst these price decreases were quite successful from the public authorities' point of view, there are some important negative spillovers. Volumes of these drugs decreased quite dramatically because there was no interest in promoting or supporting them, and generics manufacturers are still very small compared to

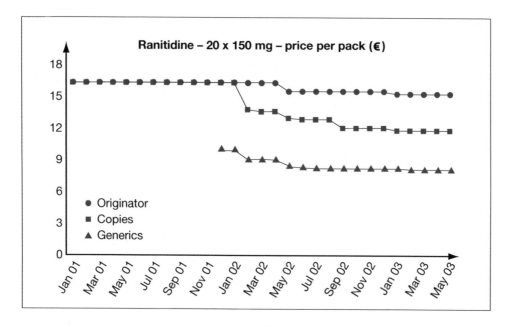

FIGURE 4.5   Price variations for ranitidine. Source: IMS data.

big pharmaceutical companies. For instance, ranitidine lost more than 30% of its volume after the generic launch.

In parallel to the development of Level I reference pricing, public authorities might again consider implementing Level II reference pricing, in order to enlarge the reference price system to include patented drugs. This would not be good news for companies, of course. Italian authorities might think about Level II reference pricing because a successful strategy for big companies has been to switch their promotional efforts with prescribers to similar products still under patent protection and which are therefore excluded from Level I reference pricing. Sale volumes of omeprazole, which will be off-patent in Italy soon, are falling. There is a delay in the date of patent expiry in Italy compared to other European countries because there has been a national, very protective, law which extended the term of patents in Italy.

Turning to the pharmacists' right of substitution in Italy, a pharmacist can substitute a cheaper equivalent drug for prescribed medicines, unless the substitution is prohibited by a physician. Generic substitution has not had a significant effect in Italy's generics market because, although important in principle, it is not relevant as pharmacists do not obtain sufficient financial incentives to support dispensing generics, unlike in other countries, such as France. Thus, the share of generics – which in Italy are semi-branded generics, that is, the name of the active principal plus the name of the brand – is still very low. For example, in 2002 expenditure on off-patent drugs and semi-branded generics represented, respectively, 7% and 1% of public pharmaceutical expenditure. In 2004, these percentages rose to 10% for off-patented drugs and nearly 2% for semi-branded generics; still very low.

National P&R policies in the future

Predicting possible future scenarios for the Italian pharmaceutical market is, for many reasons, very difficult. There are still uncertainties surrounding the contents of the latest finance bill to be passed in Italy and how this bill will be applied in practice.

At this stage, AIFA may base price negotiations for innovative medicines on their added therapeutic value. AIFA will probably set clear criteria on how to link the degree of innovation to a premium price. There are two basic issues surrounding this link that need to be taken into account. First, premium prices in Italy have so far not been given in practice, and this is an important issue for AIFA, which is seriously trying to tackle this problem, but has no experience up to date. The second issue refers to what constitutes an innovative drug, and how the degree of innovation can be assessed in practice.

On the other hand, the so-called 'me-too' drugs and new indications will be tackled in a different way. AIFA will probably move towards a more articulated price negotiation strategy, based on the full product portfolio of each company. As in other countries, and as mentioned before, the crucial issue will be what is considered to be an innovative drug and what is not. It seems that AIFA will be happy to move towards a more full-product portfolio in a 'PPRS-like' system, although it will probably not control profits but prices. Alternatively it may follow the French example.

The premium price for innovative drugs should be negotiated between companies and AIFA, on the basis of five key issues – which are easy to list but difficult to apply in practice.

1. Companies' investment in manufacturing plants – probably the easiest factor to quantify.

2. Increased R&D expenditures versus marketing activities.

3. Development of advanced clinical trials.

4. Choice of Italy as *rapporteur* country for EU approvals of innovative drugs.

5. Increase of exports and free trade of raw materials and products.

One of the concerns of the new agency, which is underlined in the third and fourth issues above, is to try to attract investment to the country by encouraging companies to conduct Phase 1 and Phase 2 clinical trials in Italy. However, this strategy may be difficult to accept in Europe. Nevertheless, there is clearly a concern, because AIFA will be funded from companies' submission fees. Here Italy is unfortunately the Cinderella again – it has seldom been chosen as the rapporteur country so far.

What are the other issues that might drive Italian pharmaceutical policy in the next 10 years? First, will Italy move towards a two-lane approach, whereby patented, innovative drugs and generics are differentiated? The answer may be 'yes', because the two lanes have been quite clear-cut, namely the patented and off-patent drugs. However, this two-lane approach could converge if enlarged therapeutic-equivalence reference price groups (i.e. Level 2) are rolled out, as has happened in Germany, the Netherlands and New Zealand.

Another issue is whether Italy moves towards a budgetary approach to control GP prescribing. This is the crucial issue in countries like Italy, France, Spain and Germany. The problem is how to put a budgetary approach into practice effectively. The devolution process means that some regions will move in this direction while others will not be able to do it. It is something which will be very difficult to detect, but it is the major challenge for pharmaceutical policy in Italy.

Discussion

Reference prices and generics

Q: You have a graph that shows how the reference price (RP) system has cut generic prices. However, I recently read about the RP in Italy and I understand that, between 1992 and 2000, the total costs of drug expenditure have gone up every year. Is this correct?

Q: My second question relates to generic substitution. Does Italy also have generic prescribing by doctors?

A: As to your first question, it is probably fair to say that in all countries pharmaceutical expenditure has increased. However, the available information on pharmaceutical expenditure across countries shows that Italy has lower increases compared to the average.

Regarding your second question, I omitted to say that all prescriptions are still written down with the branded name, so there is no generic prescribing. Generic prescribing is probably very useful to help generics. However, at the same time, generic prescribing can also create a crisis in the whole system, given the Italian system is based on the prescription of the brand name, as in Spain, France and Germany. Encouraging generic prescribing is thus another critical issue – which is not only a cultural issue but also affects business. Also there is a lot of co-marketing activity in Italy and generic prescribing, if analysed from a broader perspective, is linked ultimately to what drug is being dispensed. Hence, generic prescribing would create problems for patented drugs.

Q: So the generics are branded generics?

A: Yes. I call them 'semi-branded generics'. We also have branded generics. Branded generics are copies and they are much more important than in the UK, because they existed before generics.

Q: My comment is about generic policy and reference pricing. I think that there are two types of generic policy: one which relies on prescribers, as in the UK for instance – with 80% generic prescription – and another especially in France, which relies on generic distribution, where pharmacists are paid to distribute generics but the doctors do not care. Clearly the influence on the generic market is different according to the incentives created, either at the level of the prescribers or at the level of the distributors.

In no country is there a policy which encourages the consumer. The consumer is not better reimbursed whether he has a generic or a branded product. To my knowledge, there is no country – perhaps in the US, but not in Europe – where there is discrimination between the two.

Reference pricing may be more harmful in those countries where distribution is involved than in those where prescribers are involved. To pay for the distributors you need to have a different price, to encourage them to create an incentive. If you have a prescriber policy, it is not important that the price is different from the reimbursement price. I think that reference pricing is less important under a prescribing policy than under a distribution policy. I would like to hear your view on that.

What we support in France is the involvement of the consumer. We try to make the government sensitive to the fact that one of the problems relating to healthcare is to make the consumer more responsible. We have tried to push that idea, but it is difficult in Europe.

A: I think that you are right. You have stressed the important points. Roughly speaking, there are two ways in which to help support a generics market: to enhance prescribers or to enhance dispensers. At the beginning, our attempt was to affect prescribers, but it did not work. Now there is a more 'French' system, where dispensers should be helped – because they have the right of substitution, which is very important for a pharmacist. Thus, as in other countries, pharmacists can negotiate extra, 'hidden' discounts. We are still wondering whether or not this is legal, but it does happen. I cannot give you a precise answer to the question regarding Italy because the generics market is still very small. So far, most agents involved in the system are not very interested in generics.

At the present time, I would say that the dispenser has greater advantages in dispensing some generics. Indeed, the few generics that are dispensed are dispensed because of pharmacists. There is some information that shows there are instances where pharmacists deny they have an available generic when a patient asks for it, or that pharmacists do not ask for the co-payment if the 'copy' of the product has a price higher than the reference price because perhaps the producing company will cover it. The situation is very obscure in this sense, but it is not yet a real concern because the market is still very limited.

I fully agree with you in your assertion that patients should be involved. There is a very easy way to address the problem: exempt generics from the flat charge co-payment (the prescription charge). The patient is the most important element in terms of encouraging generics, once it is explained that they are equivalent drugs. However, if GPs undermine the reliability of generics it is easy to reverse the story. At this stage, I should mention that we have abolished co-payments and charges at a national level, although some regions have reintroduced the flat charge on prescriptions.

Measures promoting R&D

Q: I have read that AIFA is also in charge of implementing measures to promote R&D in Italy. When I read that, I could not really believe it. Looking at it from a European perspective, it seems to be a major conflict of interest: on the one hand, the agency decides on pricing and reimbursement and, on the other, it favours R&D in Italy. How is this implemented?

A: This issue is part of AIFA's remit, but it still needs to be seen how it is managed. You are right to raise the problem of a conflict of interest. I wonder what happens in other countries. However, I think that Italy's real problem is that we are the last ones who have 'boarded the train': other nations have been much more successful in doing precisely that, trying to support the domestic pharmaceutical industry.

Remuneration schemes for pharmacists

Q: It is my understanding that there is a proposal in Italy regarding a new way of paying pharmacists – or perhaps it has already been implemented – which involves a decrease in the margin for drug dispensing. Could you elaborate on that? There has also been such a proposal in Spain.

A: This would take some time to go into but I will try to summarise it. The problem is that regions realised they could not contain pharmaceutical expenditure and they would be incurring a deficit. Someone therefore suggested, 'Why not cut down the distribution margin?' The idea was to buy drugs for community care in a 'hospital-like' way; that is, to use public procurement, or tenders, to buy medicines for community care. This was successfully challenged by the regional and local associations of pharmacy owners. What happened eventually was the so-called 'double' system where, for a very limited list of drugs, public regional authorities buy drugs – or their health authorities buy them – with a discount comparable to that of hospitals; but the drugs are still distributed by pharmacies. Patients do not understand the difference, but the real difference is in some modest cost saving to the Italian NHS. Some LHAs try to stress that this saving is between 20%–30%, but that may be overestimated and is only for a limited list of drugs anyway.

References

Centro di Ricerche sulla Gestione dell'Assistenza Sanitaria e Sociale (CERGAS) (2006) *Osservatorio Farmaci.* Report no 17. CERGAS, Milan.

Garattini L and Ghislandi S (2006) Off-patent drugs in Italy: a short sighted view? *European Journal of Health Economics.* **7**: 79–83.

CHAPTER 5

Pricing and reimbursement policies in Spain: current and future trends

Joan Costa-i-Font

This chapter discusses pricing and reimbursement policies in Spain. It starts with a very brief overview of the healthcare system in Spain, followed by a more extensive overview of the pharmaceutical market. For this purpose, first is offered some information on pharmaceutical expenditure in Spain, and its main drivers, followed by a discussion of the institutional design of pharmaceutical policies in Spain. A discussion about the pricing and reimbursement system in Spain is presented, differentiating between policies aimed at the supply and demand sides, respectively. Finally, there are comments on the current policy discussion taking place in Spain. There is presently a proposal to reform the Medicines Act in Spain which, if it receives parliamentary approval, will represent a total change in the paradigm of how pharmaceutical policies are implemented.* Certain issues regarding pharmaceutical policy, such as discounting, controlling piracy and setting up a reference-pricing system, are similar to those in Italy.

---

* Note from the Editors: The Medicines Law was finally approved on 26 July 2006. Where relevant, we have added a footnote explaining whether the policies discussed by the author have been ultimately implemented, and in what form.

Overview of the healthcare system in Spain

Health policy in Spain is driven by the fact that the system is decentralised to 17 different regions. The decentralisation process started in the 1980s, when Catalonia received healthcare responsibilities. In 1985, it was Andalusia; in the 1990s, five new regions took on healthcare responsibilities and, from 2002, the whole system became fully decentralised. The former INSALUD – the agency which regulated the system and which was responsible for health policy in those regions with their responsibility still at the central level – disappeared. The Spanish National Health Service (NHS) may now be characterised as a system of health services, rather than a single health service in itself. We will see that this is an important factor driving pharmaceutical policy, especially for demand-side policies, given that pricing and reimbursement of medicines, as well as licensing, remain the responsibility of the national government.

Spain currently funds its health system on the basis of tax, although it was not until 1999 that taxes fully funded the NHS.

Overview of the Spanish pharmaceutical market

One of the main features of the Spanish pharmaceutical market is that Spain devotes €1 out of every €4 invested in healthcare to drugs. This means that medicines in Spain are seen as a high-priority input, especially in sectors such as mental health. Overall, pharmaceuticals represent 1.6% of Spanish gross domestic product (GDP).

The market for drugs in Spain is dominated by prescription medicines. However, there is a difference in terms of whether the market is measured by volume or value of sales. In value terms, prescription drugs account for 92% of total sales, while in volume terms, this percentage is lower at 85%.

Another important characteristic of the Spanish pharmaceutical market is that generic penetration is limited; in fact, it is half of the overall percentage in the European Union (EU). Generics are normally priced at a lower level than on-patent medicines. Generic medicines currently represent 7.5% and 13.8% of the total medicines market in value and volume terms, respectively. However, there has been a significant increase in the number of generic products in the market. Spain, like Italy, had a large number of copies in the market, because there was no full patent protection until 1992, when product patents were approved. From July 1993 onwards, generics started to be launched in the country. The generic market has grown steadily since then. Encouraging generic medicines is one of the main discussion points in terms of Spanish pharmaceutical policy at the present time.

Another important feature is that Spanish drug companies do not invest very much in R&D, as in other southern European countries. In fact, R&D investment seems to have declined in importance from 1987. In 1987, R&D represented 8.6% of pharmaceutical sales, while in 2001 this proportion fell to 7.9%.

The main driver of pharmaceutical expenditure in Spain seems to be the high price of new drugs and, in particular, the high cost of new treatments. The price for new drugs in Spain is in line with other European countries while the price, on average, for all drugs is far behind (*see* Kanavos *et al.*, 2004). For instance, the cost per prescription in Spain, in constant terms, was €6.69 in 1992 and €9.18 in 2002 – a significant increase.

Looking at expenditure, the fastest growing part of pharmaceutical expenditure comes as no surprise at all: it is the NHS (public) market, as shown in Figure 5.1. Figure 5.1 shows how overall pharmaceutical expenditure can be decomposed between the over-the-counter (OTC) market, the co-payment paid by the patient (termed as 'cost sharing' in the figure below) and public expenditure.

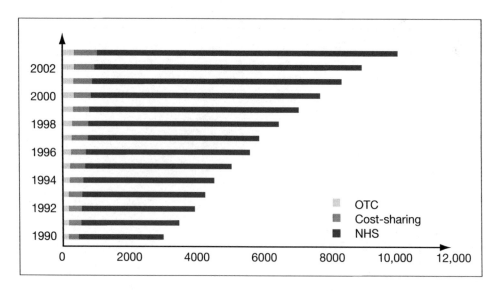

FIGURE 5.1   Pharmaceutical expenditure in Spain, 1990–2003 (€, million). Source: Spanish Ministry of Health (2005) (www.msc.es).

The drug price composition between ex-factory price, distribution margins and indirect taxation has not changed very much over the last 20 years, as shown in Figure 5.2.

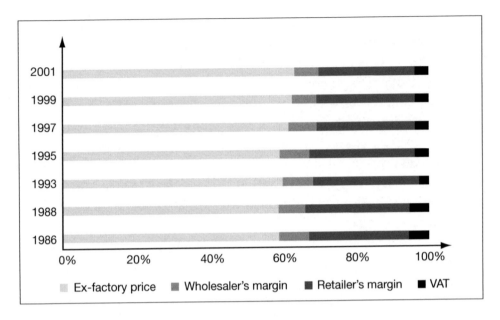

FIGURE 5.2 Price decomposition, 1986–2001. Source: Farmaindustria (2004).

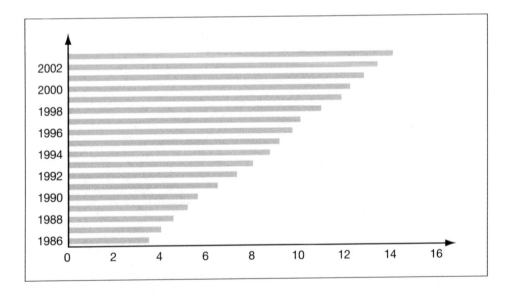

FIGURE 5.3 Cost per NHS prescription in Spain, constant terms, 1986–2003 (€).
Source: Spanish Ministry of Health (2005) (www.msc.es).

The main driver of pharmaceutical expenditure in Spain is the cost per prescription, the evolution of which is shown in Figure 5.3.

The number of prescriptions dispensed increased during the 1990s. This had to do with a number of factors. For instance, the decrease in the cost-sharing level (i.e. level of patient co-payment), the integration of GPs into the NHS system increasing the probability of visiting a doctor (which the data from the National Health Survey seem to show) and the full decentralisation process.

Now we focus on the potential existence of regional heterogeneity across the Spanish regions, especially in terms of public pharmaceutical expenditure. Figure 5.4 shows how public pharmaceutical expenditure evolved for the seven regions with devolved healthcare responsibilities prior to 2002 (Andalusia, Basque Country, Canary Islands, Catalonia, Galicia, Navarra and Valencia) compared to the rest of the regions – the INSALUD, which was the agency then responsible for health policy at the central level.

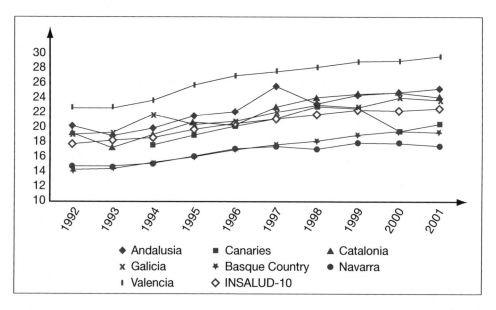

FIGURE 5.4   Regional heterogeneity in the percentage of public pharmaceutical expenditure (out of total healthcare expenditure). Source: Spanish Ministry of Health (2005) (www.msc.es).

Comparing the share of public expenditure on medicines shows there are significant differences between regions. In particular, Valencia shows a systematically higher share of public pharmaceutical expenditure out of total healthcare spending.

We now turn to the proportion of pharmaceutical expenditure borne by patients. This proportion, together with the relative importance of consumption by the elderly in Spain, is illustrated in Figure 5.5.

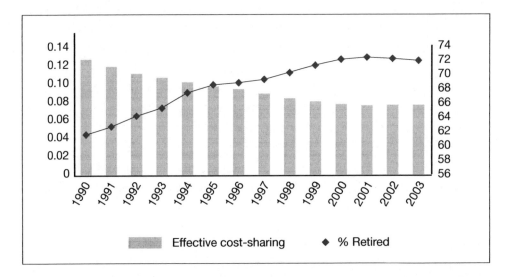

FIGURE 5.5 Cost sharing and percentage of consumption by the elderly. Source: Spanish Ministry of Health (2005) (www.msc.es).

Figure 5.5 shows how the relative importance of cost-sharing (i.e. patient co-payments) has declined since the 1990s. This trend continues that observed during the 1980s. In 1990, patient co-payment represented more than 12% of pharmaceutical expenditure but by 2003, this proportion had fallen to less than 8%. On the other hand, the share of pharmaceutical expenditure consumed by the retired population was up to 72% in 2003, from 62% in 1990. That suggests there may be some moral hazard taking place in the Spanish pharmaceutical market, given that retired people do not need to co-pay for their medicines, that is, they get their medicines for free.* Furthermore, there is evidence of some 'pirating' (or fraud) – by 'pirating' is meant that certain elderly persons who are exempt from co-payments may buy drugs for the rest of the family.

In summary, the rise in medicines' expenditure in Spain seems to be driven mainly by the rise in the cost per prescription. As discussed below, there is also some

---

* Given that the retired population is excluded from cost-sharing, there are very limited incentives to consume cheaper versions of specific products and to cut the number of prescriptions, both from the consumer and the provider sides.

possible over-reimbursement to drug distributors; here we refer to the important role of discounts, and the non-existence of claw-back mechanisms for the Ministry of Health. There has been integration of GPs within the NHS, and a devolution process has been taking place. This implies that volume is mainly determined at the regional level, while prices and reimbursement are determined at the central level. There is now some discussion on whether regions should also participate in the pricing and reimbursement – and that may be one of the things which will happen in the future.

Current trends in national P&R regulation

One of the challenges faced in the regulation of the Spanish pharmaceutical market during the 1980s and especially in the 1990s, was the 'universalisation' process. In parallel, GPs have been integrated better into the NHS, which it could be argued, has increased the probability of a patient visiting the doctor. There has also been a moderate liberalisation of the retail pharmacy sector since 1997.

A feature which Spain shares with other European countries such as Italy is that the health system is relatively decentralised. However, at the national level, there are three ministries involved in drug regulation. Patent registration is normally the responsibility of the Ministry of Industry. The Ministry of Health is in charge of the licensing process through its Directorate General of Pharmacy, although the authorisation is undertaken by the Spanish Agency for Medicines. P&R is normally the responsibility of the Treasury – the Ministry of Finance – together with the Ministry of Health. Table 5.1 shows the relevant stakeholders in Spain.

As a result of the decentralisation process in Spain, pharmaceutical policy focusing on the 'volume' variable (rather than price) is mainly the responsibility of the regions. This issue is explored further below. The co-ordination of the whole system has been the responsibility of the Inter-Territorial Commission of Regional Health Services since 2002, when the full decentralisation process took place.

As far as the industry is concerned, manufacturers, OTC producers and generic producers represent significant lobbies in terms of pharmaceutical policy in the country. Doctors – as in Germany – represent another important and influential lobby, as do pharmacists. Consumers and patients might have an important role in the future, but currently are not well organised. Scientists and trades unions are quite weak in healthcare policy.

TABLE 5.1 Institutional setting

Stakeholders	Responsibility
Drug regulation	
Product licensing	DG Pharmacy and Health Products (MoH)
Product authorisation	Spanish Agency for Medicines (MoH)
Patent registration	Ministry of Industry (MoI)
Price regulation	Interministerial Commission on Drug Prices (MoH) and Ministry of Finance (MoF)
Reimbursement	National Commission for Rational Use of Medicines
Distributors' mark-ups	Interministerial Commission on Drug Prices (MoH and MoF)
Co-ordination	Inter-Territorial Commission of Regional Health Services
Prescription and provision	Regional Department of Health
Industry	
Manufacturers	Famaindustria
OTC producers	Association of Public Medicines
Generic producers	Association of Generic Drug Producers
Other health service stakeholders	
Doctors	College of Medical Doctors
Pharmacists	College of Pharmacists
Consumers	Association of Spanish Consumers
Patients	Specific patient associations
Scientists	Specific disease scientific associations
Trades unions	Specific trades unions

OTC, over-the-counter.

Supply-side policies

P&R in Spain follows the lines of a rigid and, as in other countries, non-transparent, product-by-product regulation. It follows a sort of cost-plus system, although certain factors, such as the price of drugs in other European countries, are taken into account when setting the price for each product. But again it is important to stress the fact that the link between price and such factors is not really transparent.

Despite the fact that prices are heavily regulated, the NHS has often resorted to compulsory price reductions as a way of cutting pharmaceutical expenditure. There is plenty of evidence to show that this may have a one-year or two-year effect, but it does not really reduce prices in the long term; therefore, other instruments have been tried.

One such instrument is the use of de-listing – which could be defined as introducing a negative list. Spain has experienced the de-listing of drugs twice: in 1993 and 1998. These had a very limited effect on expenditure and some effect on product renewal (Costa-i-Font and Puig-Junoy, 2005).

There is also a generic reference-price system, implemented in the same year as in Italy (2000). The reference-price formula has already been modified three times and does not seem to be producing the expected savings, at least until the introduction of the 2005 reforms (Puig-Junoy, 2005).

The pricing of medicines is not innovation-driven, and that is probably one of the main challenges in the future. Drugs are included in the catalogue, that is, the positive list, only on the basis of product safety, efficacy and effectiveness. Cost-effectiveness is not really taken into account, although it is important to stress that it is probably one of the areas where we could expect change in the future. At the regional level there are health technology agencies – for example, in Andalusia and Catalonia – and there is a Department in the Ministry of Health that is responsible at the central level for pharmaco-economic evaluation studies, although the latter agency does not focus specifically on medicines. In the future, there will probably be an agency at the national level, with its main focus being to look more formally at economic (i.e. cost-effectiveness) data – but it is too early to know how this agency will work.

Cost containment has not been a priority. In addition, it is probably useful to recall that Spain was under a dictatorship 30 years ago. Public expenditure in the 1970s was about 25% of the GDP, so the main priority at the time was to modernise the country and to set up a universal system. The system was therefore transformed from being social insurance based to tax-funded.

Generic penetration has not been a priority either. An important area of discussion in Spain has been the expansion of hospital consumption. It is also important to stress that there are limited provider incentives. GPs are paid on a salary basis and there is no capitation adjustment. There have been some experiments with budgets, which will be discussed later, and dispensers are paid on the basis of a proportional mark-up, which fosters the dispensing of high-price drugs rather than supporting efficiency objectives.

On the supply side the two main supporting policies have been the reference-price system and the de-listings.

The reference-price system was set up in December 2000, and was introduced by the Conservative government. It involved only 98 product categories. At the time, the reference price was calculated as a weighted average of the three lowest-priced products, which represented at least 20% of the total market within a group. The main problem of the system was that it had limited incentives for price reductions. In fact, it led to an increase in the price for those products that were cheaper than the reference price, and there was a very limited price reduction of those products which were above the reference price.

In 2002 there was an adjustment of the reference price system. New groups were included, but it still suffered from the same limitations. In 2003, a further reform, called the 'Quality and Cohesion Law', included a new reference-price system. This time, the reference price was based on the three lowest costs of the treatments, adjusted by defined daily dose (DDD).

One of the main problems with the reference price system was that it fostered the use of discounts – an endemic problem in the Spanish pharmaceutical market – as well as the prescription of high-dosage drugs. Partly because this system was introduced by the Conservative government, it is being reformed under the future new Medicines Act by the current Socialist government. The new reference price will be calculated on the basis of the three lowest prices of the products within a drug category.

One of the main changes introduced by the future Medicines Act, if approved in its November 2005 form, is that all branded medicines that have been in the Spanish market for 10 years and for whatever reason have no generic competitor in the Spanish market but have a generic version in any EU country, will have their price reduced by 20%. This has been a highly controversial issue. In addition, whilst the current regulation seems to include the prohibition of price discounts (although not explicitly), the version of the Medicines Bill, as of November 2005, makes this prohibition explicit.

With regard to measures, implemented at national level, aimed at controlling volume, there have been two de-listing experiences. One was in 1993, when about 1700 products were de-listed. The products were about 10 years old and, because no single group was de-listed, there was simply substitution amongst products within a group. There was no evidence of any effect on expenditure. The de-listing in 1998 affected about 800 products. In this case it was even less effective than before, because it just de-listed very old products. Again, it had no effect on expenditure.

Regardless of the two de-listing experiences, the market for OTCs did not seem to develop. It may be surprising, but it seems to have declined. It was about 15% of the total medicines market in the 1980s and it is now about 6% or 7%.

Demand-side policies

Turning now to the demand-side policies, there are very mild incentives to control demand for medicines. GPs are paid on a salary basis; there is no capitation adjustment. There has been some experience with budgets, which basically give economic incentives for generic prescribing. However, it is not enough to prescribe generics, but rather there is a need to prescribe low-price generics. There is significant price variability between generics. Furthermore, some clinical guidelines are being elaborated, which is probably enhancing and improving the quality of prescribing.

Information policy is limited. For instance, in 2004, about 30% of the population did not know what a generic drug was. Another important feature to bear in mind is that there has not been a reform of the cost-sharing system for 20 years. This could be an example of 'non-decision making'. Over the last 20 years Spain has not changed co-payments, which gives medicines free of charge to individuals once they retire. The general population pays 40% of the retail price, while disabled patients pay 10%. This translates into a significant reduction in cost-sharing from the 1980s to 2003. In 1985, 15% of total NHS expenditure was paid by the patients themselves. In 2003, the share had dropped to 6.8%. There is no political consensus regarding any reform of co-payment levels, because the retired population is about 20% of the total population and such a move would, in electoral terms, be strongly penalised by voters and their families.

Thanks to the decentralisation process, innovations in the way pharmaceuticals are regulated in Spain have been introduced at regional level. For example, Andalusia introduced in 2001 prescription by International Nonproprietary Names (INN) – although this decision might be partly due to the fact that Andalusia had a Socialist government and at that time the central government was Conservative. Andalusia also introduced some modifications to the national reference price system for its region, which meant that the reference price in Andalusia was about 7% to 10% lower than the reference price in the rest of the country. It has had a high level of acceptance amongst GPs and it has also produced sizeable savings. In that case, therefore, decentralisation seems to have had an effect.

Turning to the distributors and dispensers, drug distribution in Spain shows very mild evidence of competition. There is a stable number of pharmacists and wholesalers. For instance, the number of pharmacists per 1000 inhabitants has been relatively stable at around 0.45–0.50 since the late 1980s. It is interesting to note that the wholesale business is vertically integrated with pharmacists' business; indeed, 70% of wholesalers are co-operatives of pharmacists.

One of the key issues of demand-side policy in Spain refers to the way dispensers are paid. As mentioned before, the financing of drug dispensing was based on a linear tariff. It was a linear margin, as in other countries – 9.6% for wholesalers and 27.7% for retailers – and it is well-known that this kind of system fosters the dispensing of high-price drugs. The margins allowed in the distribution system were changed in 2000, when a form of non-linear tariff was introduced. When the price of the medicine exceeds the threshold of €78 at ex-factory level, the mark-up is fixed at €8.54 and €33.54 for wholesalers and pharmacists, respectively; hence, in theory, there is no incentive to continue dispensing high-price drugs. In 2005, the threshold and mark-ups were updated – the threshold increased from €78 to €89.63, while the fixed mark-up was increased to €37.53 for the retailer and decreased to €7.37 for the wholesaler.

The problem in the pharmacist sector is the role played by discounts. Regardless of the reform in the way pharmacists are paid, pharmacists receive large discounts. Unlike in the UK, there is no way that the NHS can claw back any savings generated by the discount. Most discounts are quantity discounts rather than price discounts, so they are totally non-transparent.

There is currently a discussion in Spain regarding the way pharmacists are paid. Spain is now trying to introduce a decreasing margin on the basis of sales. This could produce some effect, especially if the non-linear tariff that was introduced in 2000 is maintained.

Recent changes in P&R regulation

As mentioned before, there is currently a reform of the general Medicines Act in Spain. Three main issues are being discussed at present. It could be the case that none of them are finally introduced in the new Law, but given the attention they are receiving, they merit some discussion here.

The first main issue is a 20% reduction of drug prices after 10 years of product authorisation for a drug in Spain when this product has no generic in the market – as long as there is a generic drug in another European country. As I see it, this regulation could ultimately expand the generics market in Spain but, at the same time, it could reduce the incentives to enter strategically in different European countries. There are arguments being made against this piece of regulation. One comes from the Ministry of Industry, arguing that the price reductions of such products should be gradually implemented; the Treasury agrees that it should be case by case. On the other hand, the Council of State – a sort of internal advisory committee aimed at balancing the opinion of the government – argues that in any case the price should not fall below the price of the generic in these other countries of reference, plus a reasonable mark-up.

The second main issue under discussion in Spain – and why I think there is now a change in the paradigm in the way pharmaceutical policy is being implemented – is the tax imposed on pharmaceutical companies on their total drug sales, ranging between 1.5% and 5% of sales. The problem with the way this tax is designed is that it reduces the advantage from company concentration. The Council of State also argues that the percentages are far too large, and suggests that these rebates should be implemented on a case-by-case basis rather than as a general rule. If this were to be the case, it would probably lead to considerable lobbying.

The third issue under discussion is the banning of discounts and, indirectly, the banning of parallel trade. It seems that price discounts will be considered illegal and prosecuted, through both formal and informal mechanisms – the latter being something like information systems. However, the Council of State argues that quantity discounts and early payment discounts should be maintained. If that were to be so, it would undermine the entire regulation, because the vast majority of discounts that take place are transport and quantity discounts.*

Also currently under discussion is the requirement for manufacturers, wholesalers and retailers to report the price at which they sell each drug. This is an indirect way of controlling parallel trade because if manufacturers know the price at which the drug will be sold then they could implement a 'double or dual' pricing approach. In any case, the whole system would become more transparent and, indirectly, less profitable.

---

* Note from the Editors: The first issue (20% price cut) was finally implemented, as well as the tax on sales. However, the approved tax rates were 1.5% for quarterly sales (at ex-factory price) of up to three million euros, and 2% for quarterly sales above three million euros. Also, discounts have been explicitly prohibited, although quantity discounts and early payment discounts are allowed – although these have to be transparent.

National P&R policies in the future

To conclude, I will offer some thoughts which may help to ascertain what future scenarios could be possible for the Spanish pharmaceutical market.

First, there is evidence of regulatory failure in the Spanish pharmaceutical sector. Not only is there evidence of this failure, but also there is great frustration among policymakers with regard to the regulation of the pharmaceutical industry.

It seems that the new pharmaceutical bill will deal with the lack of transparency in the way medicines are regulated in Spain. If the issues currently under discussion are implemented, there will be a reduced incentive for company concentration. There will be a reduction, or at least a moderation, in the price of new treatments. There may be some increase in the penetration of generic drugs. We could also expect a reduction of parallel trade. Those who have any interest in distributing drugs in Spain will not be too pleased with the changes, because there will probably be tighter controls on the way distributors are paid. In addition, reform of cost-sharing mechanisms could be included, but this necessarily requires a political agreement.

Discussion

Parallel trade and the distribution market

Q: Related to your comments on parallel trade, are we talking about discouraging parallel export here?

A: Yes.

Q: What is the policy issue for the government? If there is a lot of parallel trade out of Spain, does it mean that potentially companies are looking for higher prices in Spain to stop it happening?

A: The problem is shortages. At least, that is what is formally under discussion. There is evidence that in certain areas there have occasionally been shortages, which could be due to parallel trade. On the other hand, at the LSE we have carried out some studies on the parallel trade issue and it seems that Spain is becoming the clear-cut substitute for France as a parallel exporter. It provides additional evidence that preventing parallel trade in indirect ways could be efficient.

Q: Continuing with the same issue, I have doubts about why national authorities should struggle against parallel trade in a country where there are parallel exports. This is also quite clearly supported by the EU. I know there is the matter of the so-called 'quotas', because a lot of companies try to restrict their production – but I do not understand why the public authorities should be involved in this matter in such a clear-cut way.

Q: Second, you have spoken about discounts. I suppose you mean extra discounts kept by pharmacists. Is that correct?

A: Yes.

Q: As you know, it is quite a grey area and difficult to detect. I wonder how you can really detect these extra discounts, because there is trade everywhere. It may be a nice idea in principle, but in practice I wonder how public authorities would be able to detect this problem – which has been a problem everywhere and very unsuccessfully detected.

A: One of the problems of the wholesale system in Spain is that there are wholesalers specialised in parallel trade. That being the case, certain drugs that are being distributed by certain specialised wholesalers may not go to the right place and may be diverted to another European country. That is something which the public authorities should prevent, or at least regulate.

It is not only the issue of discounts that is of importance and without an easy solution. Some movement towards the introduction of information controls in relation to distributors – who are the ones who have benefited most from a non-transparent system – could, as a signal, prevent these things happening to a certain extent. They could at least lead to the introduction of more complex ways of setting up discounts. It may be that, the more you regulate, the more sophisticated the business becomes and there is a never-ending process. As a way of signalling to distributors that something is going wrong, it could at least have some effect.

Q: I wondered why you did not mention 'Article 100' in this regard, where the pharmaceutical industry now has the flexibility to have higher prices for the products which are not being reimbursed in Spain alone. In essence, Article 100 in Spain (which has been in place for the past five years) allows price controls only on prescribed products which are reimbursed in Spain. The industry is therefore able to have higher prices, or free prices, for those products exported to other countries. That was the idea behind having this kind of dual pricing in Spain.

A: The problem is that the dual price, as you probably know, was the cause of a decision by the European Court of Justice and was at that time considered to be anticompetitive. The new regulation, which just deals with information rather than explicitly establishing dual pricing, does not seem to be anti-competitive itself. It deals with an increase in the transparency of the pharmaceutical market – at least that is the objective – rather than with explicitly banning parallel trade. There is no explicit recognition by the Spanish state that they want to abandon parallel trade, but that is probably what everyone has in mind when they read that regulation.

References

Costa-i-Font J and Puig-Junoy J (2005) Regulatory Ambivalence and the Limitations of Pharmaceutical Policy in Spain. Economics Working Paper 762. Working Paper No. 42. Research Centre on Health and Economics (CRES), University Pompeu Fabra, Barcelona.

Farmaindustria (2004). *La Industria Farmacéutica en Cifras* (The Pharmaceutical Industry in Figures). Farmaindustria, Madrid.

Kanavos P, Costa-i-Font J, Merkur S and Gemmill M (2004) *The Economic Impact of Pharmaceutical Parallel Trade in European Union Member States: A Stakeholder Analysis.* LSE Health and Social Care, London School of Economics and Political Science, London.

Puig-Junoy J (2005) *The Impact of Generic Reference Pricing Interventions in the Statin Market. Economics Working Paper 906.* Working Paper No. 48. Research Centre on Health and Economics (CRES), University Pompeu Fabra, Barcelona.

Spanish Ministry of Health (www.msc.es).

CHAPTER 6

Overview

Patricia Danzon

Introduction

The preceding chapters have provided details of the different regulatory systems currently in place and likely to develop in major European markets. In this chapter, I will present the results of some studies conducted by myself and colleagues in order to show evidence of the effects of these different policies on a number of variables.

Differential pricing versus uniform pricing

When we look at different regulatory systems from a normative or policy perspective, most economists would agree that there is fundamentally a very strong case for trying to retain systems that permit differential pricing for medicines across countries worldwide.

There are two reasons for this. First, 'static efficiency': if prices for existing drugs are different in different countries, and presumably lower in lower-income countries, this enables lower-income countries to have broader access and greater use of drugs that could not be affordable at the prices paid in high-income countries.

Second, and from a 'dynamic efficiency' standpoint, given that R&D is a global common good that has to be financed by a margin over marginal costs (in all countries combined), differential pricing indicates how different countries should contribute to the cost of R&D.

The Ramsey pricing solution to this problem is that global social welfare is maximised if prices differ across markets by a mark-up over marginal costs that is related inversely to the price elasticities of demand, if we assume everybody counts equally, that is, we do not care whether we are, for instance, French, German or English.

In theory we are trying to measure true price elasticities of demand. Actual price elasticities are very much influenced by insurance, particularly in markets where there is essentially zero co-pay, or co-pay that is insensitive to the price. A widely growing consensus therefore is that differential pricing should be based on differences in income.

This is probably not particularly relevant for the five big European countries, which show similar average per capita income. However, if we consider the new countries joining the European Union (EU), or think more broadly to developing countries, and also the US compared to other countries, then this point about maintaining differential pricing and using regulatory systems that enable differential pricing to persist is an important one.

International price comparisons

Limitations of available data

There have been a large number of studies providing cross-national price comparisons. However, they have reached similar conclusions with different degrees of precision and accuracy. This is due to a number of factors. First, when undertaking international price comparisons with the purpose of trying to evaluate the effects of different regulatory systems, we need a broad representative market basket of the products used in the countries concerned. As the market baskets vary significantly across countries, this can be very difficult. Not only do the compounds differ but, for given compounds, the formulations, the strengths and the pack sizes are different. In order to do an 'apples-to-apples' comparison, one can use only a very small fraction of the market to perform the comparison. For this reason most of the studies that have been undertaken:

▸ compare only the prices of on-patent branded drugs

▸ usually look at one pack per product

- do not weight for utilisation, which differs significantly across countries
- often consider the retail prices, which are influenced by the distribution margins, rather than the manufacturers' prices
- ignore off-invoice manufacturer discounts, for which it is very difficult to get information.

Price and availability of pharmaceuticals: evidence from nine countries

This section reports the results from a study we did using Intercontinental Medical Statistics (IMS) data for 249 leading molecules (by volume) in the US in 1999 (Danzon and Furukawa, 2003). We are in the process of updating this study using current data. To date, qualitatively, the results obtained have been similar to the previous analysis, at least among the European countries considered here – the exception being that the US is probably relatively higher-priced now.

The results from this study are interesting in that they are somewhat different from conventional wisdom. The analysis considers all products in each compound or molecule, that is, both brands and generics; manufacturer-level prices; and adjusts for off-invoice discounts in the US, where manufacturers very commonly offer discounts on the on-patent products to the managed-care companies and to the government.

The aim of the study was to compare average drug prices in the US with those in eight other countries: Canada, Chile, France, Germany, Italy, Japan, Mexico and the UK. We obtained a US-based market basket intended to include the most frequently used drugs in the US and calculated the price indices using US volume weights. On this basis, we found that our sample represents around 61% of sales in the US, the UK and Canada – so a very similar percentage in those countries – but only 30% to 40% of sales in the other countries.

The structure of the markets in the countries considered is quite dissimilar. As I mentioned before, the main discrepancy is due to differences in the presentations. This is shown by the fact that requiring a match presentation by presentation (i.e. tablet of a given strength) cuts in half the sample size that can be used and thus leads to a very unrepresentative comparison. In the results that I will be reporting, therefore, we used a comparison based on molecules, which are the same in each country.

Figure 6.1 shows the differences in the market structure between branded and unbranded generics in volume and sales terms. On the one hand, unbranded generics represent 44% of the US market in volume terms, although they account

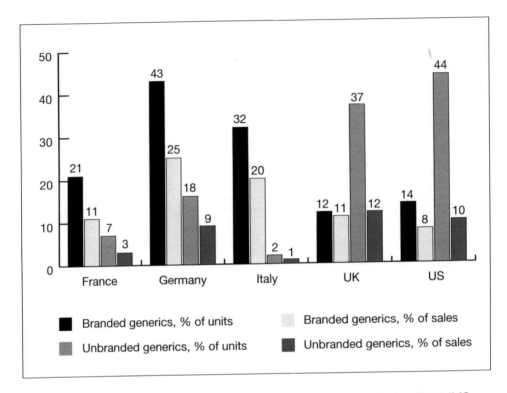

FIGURE 6.1   Branded versus unbranded generics share of unit and sales (1999 IMS data). Source: Danzon and Furukawa (2003).

for only 10% in value. Unbranded generics, which do not try to preserve and promote a brand image, only compete on price. Indeed, the cheapest generics dominate the generic market in the US – and in the UK, too.

Thus, nearly half of the US market, in volume terms, corresponds to unbranded generics, which are very cheap. By contrast, if you look at, say, France or even Germany, most of the generics are branded generics and the difference between the per cent of sales and per cent of volume is not so stark – meaning the generics are relatively more expensive compared to on-patent medicines than in the US.

Overall price indices, which include both generics and the branded products, and are converted from currencies to US dollars using exchange rates, are compared. In this way, we can compare the price of the US market basket, at foreign prices relative to US prices. For example, if France is at 70% it means the US market basket would cost 30% less than it actually does in the US, if the US was to pay French prices. The differences between the US and other countries' prices in our study are significant (i.e. 20% to 30%), but they are not as large as many of those that we have seen in other studies. However, it is important to emphasise that we are considering the US market basket and using the US as a base, so everything is normalised to the US being equal to 100. For example, our results show that Canada is 33% lower than the US but if we use Canada as a base, the US would be 50% higher than Canada. It therefore makes a difference which country we use as a base.

Figure 6.2 separates the price indexes of on-patent originator products and those relative to generics, using the US as the base country.

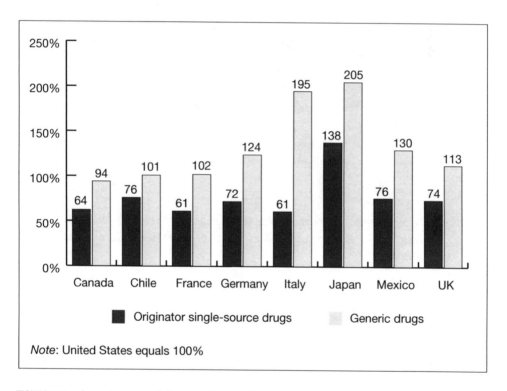

FIGURE 6.2   In-patent medicines and generics price indexes, US = 100. Source: Danzon and Furukawa (2003).

Figure 6.2 shows that, not surprisingly, the European countries – and most countries except Japan – look cheaper relative to the US when we focus on the on-patent branded products. However, when we look at the generics, all the countries included in the analysis, with the exception of Canada, have generics that are more expensive than the US generics.

The difference in market structures between the nine countries is that the US has high prices for on-patent originator drugs, but a very large market share and

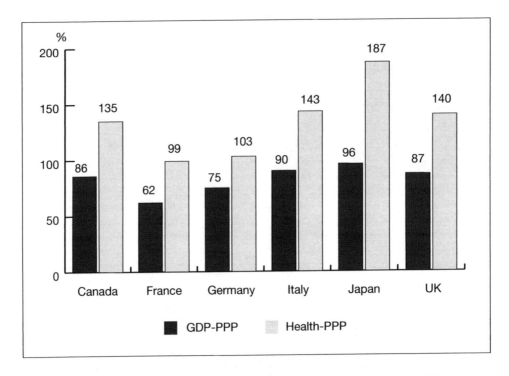

FIGURE 6.3 Comprehensive price indexes using Gross Domestic Product (GDP) Purchasing Power Parities (PPPs) and medical PPPs. Source: Danzon and Furukawa (2003).

very low prices for the off-patent, unbranded generics. On the other hand, the prices for generics tend to be relatively high in the regulated European markets. Moreover, they may well have come down since 1999 – I think that is one area where the difference of six years is probably important.

For international comparisons focusing on cost to consumers, conversion of foreign currencies at purchasing power parities (PPPs) is preferable, as exchange rates reflect the market of traded goods and also financial flows rather than the mix of goods and services that consumers buy. We used both the GDP and the medical PPPs from the OECD. The former reflects the economy-wide cost-of-living. The latter is based on the cost of purchasing a market basket of medical services, defined as a hospital stay or a physician visit, for example.

Focusing on the GDP-PPP price indexes, Figure 6.3 indicates that the differences between the foreign countries – foreign relative to the US – and the US are in several countries no longer as stark. When health PPPs are used, all countries' drugs, except France's, look more expensive than the US's. This means that prices for physicians' and hospital services in the other countries are even lower compared to the US than for drug prices. Stated in a different way, the US prices for hospital and physicians' services are even higher relative to the prices for those same services in other countries than the differential in drugs.

Nevertheless, caution should be used when considering these results, as the medical PPPs used in the analysis are not quality-adjusted. Hence, it does not take account of differences in the medical services offered in different countries (e.g. what you get in a hospital stay in the US is very different from a hospital stay in, say, the UK). However, it does make the point that the difference in drug prices is to some extent mirrored in the difference in medical service prices.

Finally, we adjusted the price differentials for the differences in average per capita income. We simply divided the price ratio by the differences in incomes. The results obtained show that most of the indexes are at or above 100 – which says that the difference in drug prices at this point in time could largely be explained by the income differences. I suspect that this would not be as true now, but this was the case in 1999.

It leaves the somewhat interesting puzzle that to some extent the differences in price of the industrialised countries mirror income differences with the exception of the two middle-income countries – Mexico and Chile – where the prices are way out of line relative to per capita income. This reflects, in particular for Mexico, the sensitivity to the comparison with the US market, but also the fact that prices in both of those countries are being set for a small, very high-income sub-group of the population, present in both those countries.

Effects of price regulation on launch of new medicines

The presence of parallel trade, which is permitted within the EU, and referencing to lower foreign prices, which is the formal basis of regulation in countries such as Italy, the Netherlands and Spain, create problems for manufacturers trying to practise differential pricing. When there are price spill-overs the rational pricing strategy is to set a uniform price, based on a weighted average of the elasticities in the different markets – where the weights reflect the relative volume shares in the different countries. Not surprisingly, with the growth of spill-overs between the European markets, there has been a movement towards greater harmony in launch prices in the EU and greater willingness of companies to delay launch, or not launch at all, if launching at a low price in a low-priced country, so as to avoid undermining the prices they obtain in higher-priced countries.

New chemical entities launch delays

To study the effects of this, we analysed the launch of 85 new chemical entities (NCEs) in the 1994–1999 period (Danzon *et al.*, 2005). We looked at the launch practices in 14 EU countries plus Australia, Canada, Czech Republic, Japan, Mexico, New Zealand, Norway, Poland, South Africa, Switzerland and the US. Using IMS data on prices and volumes, we examined the effects of the expected price – defined as the price of the drugs already on the market in the same therapeutic category – on the launch probability and delay, controlling for the market size and average per capita income.

The basic finding was that, in about half of the product/country combinations that the potential launch could have occurred, they did occur. The greatest number of launches took place in the countries that had uncontrolled prices, that is, US (73), Germany (66) and the UK (64). The fewest launches were in Japan (13), Portugal (26) and New Zealand (28). It should be noted that Japan is an outlier because it had the lowest number of launches despite its relatively high prices. The issue in Japan is not the level of prices but requirements for special trials on Japanese subjects and other regulatory delays.

In general, we found that:

▶ countries with lower prices have longer launch lags and fewer launches

▶ EU countries which are major parallel exporters have longer launch delays, controlling for expected price and volume in those countries.

Figure 6.4 shows the predicted cumulative launch probability over months since global launch.

The horizontal axis in Figure 6.4 measures months since global launch of the compound; the vertical axis reports the cumulative probability of launch. The top line is the US; the next two lines are Germany and the UK; the next three are Spain, France and Italy – countries that are fairly large markets but with regulated prices. They are followed by Portugal, which has regulated prices and is a very small market. This suggests that one of the effects of price regulation is to slow down and reduce the launch of new products.

After controlling for price and volume, we estimated the country-fixed effects, measured relative to the UK. In Figure 6.5 the UK is set at 100. The difference

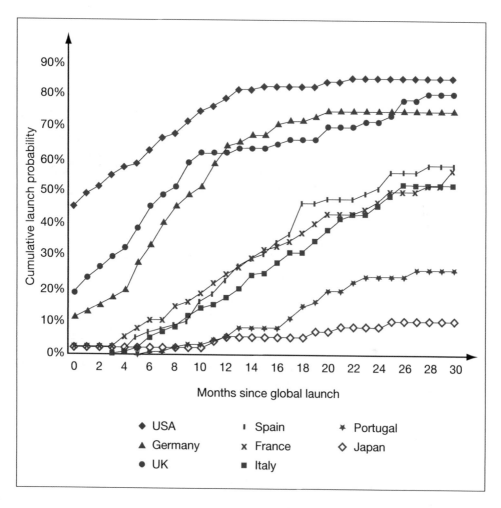

FIGURE 6.4 Kaplan–Meier estimates of cumulative launch probability for selected countries. Source: Danzon *et al.* (2005).

between the bars and 100 is the lower probability in these countries of a drug being launched, relative to the UK. From this graph it is possible to see that some of the parallel export countries – Italy, France, Belgium, Spain and Greece – have significantly lower launch probabilities.

This study, therefore, certainly found evidence of launch delays. However, we are not able to assess how much of it is due to the bureaucratic process of negotiating prices versus the strategic behaviour of companies in deciding not to launch in a low-price market because of the potential spill-over effect.

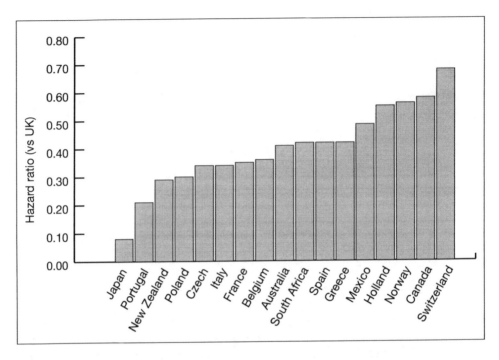

FIGURE 6.5 Countries with significantly longer delays or fewer launches, relative to the UK, controlling for price and volume.

Prices and launch probabilities: a more recent study

At the International Health Economics Association (iHEA) meeting in July 2005, we presented a study looking at a smaller set of drugs and a smaller set of countries but with more detailed data on the prices in different countries. The purpose of the study was to measure more precisely the effect of prices in different countries on launch probabilities. We found that the fact that a drug has already been launched in a high-price EU country has an effect on the launch probability in a lower-price country. The high-price countries were Germany, the Netherlands, the UK and Sweden. The lower-price countries included Spain, Italy, France and Belgium. Once a drug has been launched in a higher-price country, it increases the probability of launch in a lower-price country. That does suggest that launch delays are partly due to strategic behaviour and not just bureaucratic lag.

This study also looked at the actual launch prices, conditional on launch. We observed a significant positive relationship between the launch price of new drugs and the prices of the existing products in the market, which suggests that there is some competitive or regulatory effect on new prices. We found that there is a significant premium for the first and the second drugs in a class, where a class is defined as the therapeutic category. The first in class gets a 27% premium; the second in class gets a 17% premium; and after that it drops off.

This study therefore provides some evidence of competition in launch prices, where the follow-on products come in at lower prices in order to penetrate a market. We considered an average across all these countries, so we were not able to distinguish whether and how much this is a regulatory as opposed to a competitive effect.

Final remarks

Pricing for on-patent brands

There are two basic approaches for setting the prices of on-patent branded products. One is external referencing to the price of the same product in other countries, which applies for example in Spain and the Netherlands. The advantages of such a system are threefold: objectivity, transparency and prevention of price discrimination. However, this system is not based on the country-specific value of the drug and undermines cross-national differential pricing. This undermining of differential pricing may not be so important between the big markets of the EU. However, it plays an important role between the new accession countries and the older, higher-income EU members.

In addition, if the higher-income countries do reference the lower-price markets, there will be an external spill-over effect, which contributes to launch delays/non-launch in low-price countries and therefore reduces access to drugs in those markets. It follows that external referencing, if used, should apply between countries of similar income levels.

The other approach, which should be preferred to external referencing, is the internal benchmarking to competitor products in the same country. Within this regulatory system used in a number of countries such as France, prices of new products are set on the basis of the prices of existing compounds – competitive products in the same market – with mark-ups for innovation, preferably based on some sort of cost-effectiveness analysis rather than a flat reference pricing scheme that simply gives the same reimbursement to all the products included in a therapeutic category. Possible risks associated with this approach include lack of transparency and long price negotiations. However, it is important to emphasise that this approach has the advantage of fixing the prices of new drugs according to their value to consumers and their cost-effectiveness, and therefore can create better incentives for R&D than strict reference pricing.

Maximising savings in the generic sector

In this section I draw up a list of necessary conditions for having a competitive generic market and highlight key features in this regard of US and European regulatory systems.

First, the generics must show bio-equivalence to the originator drug through the regulatory process in order to increase the willingness of consumers and physicians to substitute generics.

Second, pharmacists must be able to substitute, unless the physician requires the brand.

Third, generic prices should be unregulated, as the regulation of generic prices tends to create a floor rather than a ceiling price and stops competition below the regulated price. Reimbursement should be based on a reference price for the molecule, usually a low-price generic in the group, and patients should pay the difference if they prefer a product with a price exceeding the reference price. This applies in the US, where there is a fixed reimbursement – called a 'maximum allowable charge' – applying to all the off-patent products in a compound and the patient pays the excess if he wants the brand product.

Finally, pharmacists should be reimbursed at a fixed dispensing fee. The incentive for the generic companies is to compete on the price at which they sell to the pharmacies, because by offering a larger margin to the pharmacy they are more likely to get the business and gain market share. In this context, the payers have to revise down the reference price over time, based on the actual acquisition prices paid by the pharmacists.

But how can third-party payers obtain reliable figures of actual discounted prices at which pharmacists buy generic products? I think it is a question of political will: being able to require that the pharmacists report what their acquisition prices are, or companies reporting the prices at which they sell, and to have significant penalties for fraudulent reporting. The US now requires the reporting of average sales price and average manufacturer price. It is confidential but there are very strict penalties for false reporting.

If the conditions indicated above are met, generic competition should work very well, as generics can compete for business and the payers capture the savings, as long as they revise down the reimbursement price. In this sort of system I would argue that discounting is not something evil, something to be got rid of; rather, it is something to take advantage of.

This is the way it works in the US, where generics gain 80% of volume once a patent expires and compete on price, leading to very low prices. Similarly, in the UK, the NHS captures savings from generic competition through the 'claw-back' system.

Conversely, in Germany generic products have relatively high prices and a large share of the market, with a predominant role for branded generics. Until 2003, pharmacies were not authorised to substitute and were paid a percentage of the medicine's price. This resulted in a market where generic products were promoted and competed on brand more than on price. Since 2003, pharmacies have been allowed to substitute and are paid a fixed fee per prescription plus a small percentage of the price.

In France, generics products, which are mostly branded generics, have a small market share. Pharmacies are traditionally not authorised to substitute and are paid a margin of the price. In 2003, a number of incentives for generic prescribing were introduced.

Discussion

Bio-equivalence of generics

Q: You said that generics must show bio-equivalence with respect to originator drugs. As it is quite a general statement, can you comment on that?

A: In the US, when the originator product expires, the generics seek approval by showing they have the same chemical composition as the originator and that they are bio-equivalent, in the sense that the level of the active ingredient in the blood is plus or minus 20% of the level that it would be with the originator product in a certain period of time from when the drug is taken.

Bio-equivalence is therefore a measure of the uptake and the stability in the bloodstream of the generic substance, and it is a measure of the clinical equivalence of the generic product to the originator product, which is very important for patients and physicians to be comfortable with generic substitution. If they are not assured that the generics really are the same as the originator products, then there is not the same willingness to substitute and you do not get the aggressive price competition.

In the Latin American markets for example, there are, as in Spain, a lot of copy products, but only some of them are bio-equivalent authorised generics. There is no general confidence in the generics, and so paying of premiums for the branded products is frequent, even once the patents have expired. In the US, once the patent has expired, everyone knows that the generics are bio-equivalent; the branded share falls to less than 20% of the market within about a year, and the generics basically take over.

Q: In Europe, it is not compulsory to demonstrate bio-equivalence. However, I think that the problem is not bio-equivalence during trials but rather in daily consumption. Public authorities should focus on the manufacturing quality and undertake controls on a regular basis.

A: I absolutely agree. I took control of manufacturing quality for granted.

Maximising saving in the generic sector. Is this possible in Europe?

Q: You presented the key characteristics of a regulatory framework which aims at lowering generics prices but can these apply to the European healthcare systems? For example, in Germany we used to believe that generic prices should be unregulated. Now, the government may need to regulate them because they are too high. You said that the payers revise reference prices and they are competing for lower prices. They are not competing for lower prices in our systems, where you have monopoly payers. The payers cannot influence the prices very much if, on the one hand, you have full coverage and, on the other, there are no direct negotiations between payers and the suppliers of health services. My question therefore is does this framework make sense in a European context?

A: I would say that the framework I described is not unique to the US, as it is very similar to what is happening in the UK now. The example of Germany, where policy-makers want to regulate the generic prices because they are too high, comes about precisely because the pharmacists have traditionally been paid a percentage margin, which creates an incentive for the pharmacists to prefer the more expensive products. In this context, generics do not compete on price but they compete on quality and brand image. Once you switch to a system where the pharmacist is paid a fixed dispensing fee, independent of the price, and can capture a margin between the reimbursement price and its acquisition cost, then the optimal strategy for generic companies is to compete on price. Then policy-makers do not need to regulate prices.

Canada is another case in point, where they have regulated the generic prices, which gravitate towards the regulated prices. Companies also give hidden discounts to the pharmacies to get their business and therefore the payers do not benefit from these savings.

For the government, in order to get the savings from the system, they need to take advantage of the competition between the generic companies which bid down the prices. Then it can revise the reimbursement price down to take advantage of the lower acquisition costs.

Since 2003, German pharmacies have been paid a fixed dispensing fee plus a percentage margin of 3%, which might seem insignificant. Whether that will be enough, who knows? I would say that it is less important to regulate the generic prices once you have a fixed dispensing fee, because then the incentive to dispense the higher-priced products would be significantly reduced.

The use of cost-effectiveness evidence in P&R procedures

COMMENT 1

We continue to get greater clarity on across-the-board price regulation, reimbursement regulation and access regulation, and yet not much clarification on the upside of providing data to support the value of your products. Where we end up, therefore, is a situation where we try to boost research within the industry to prevent or mitigate risk but we have little evidence on any upside of providing evidence. It would be interesting to know whether or not continued investment in cost-effectiveness research is producing a significant impact on payers' decisions, which ultimately affect access to our drugs for patients.

COMMENT 2

This is an important issue: what is the mechanism by which you have premiums for innovation, when is that appropriate? Patricia said that generally you need a way of getting some cost-effectiveness criteria into that. In the UK we have a mechanism. There is a mechanism in Germany controlled by IQWiG but it seems the reference groups system does not include those criteria. Also, from what Professor Graf von der Schulenburg was saying, it is very unclear whether IQWiG will do an efficient job in looking at the cost-effectiveness of those products that are not in the reference groups.

For the other countries, particularly Italy and Spain, cost-effectiveness does not seem to be playing much of a role at all in the processes. One therefore gets the sense that that part of the mechanism is what seems to be missing at the moment. Reference pricing mechanisms are in place for grouping things together and either pretending there are not any differences or refusing to pay for those differences. What we seem to be less clear about within Europe are the mechanisms for identifying whether or not there are differences, and mechanisms by which the healthcare system will pay premiums where there are differences that are valuable.

COMMENT 3

The mechanism that does what you require to be done, which is to identify value, is the market. Unfortunately, we are not very close to having access to a market in this particular sphere. Hence the question should be formulated in this way: is the investment in cost-effectiveness actually paying off in terms of delivering better access for patients to new medicines?

The root of that problem is the different motivations for conducting that work. The reason that pharmaceutical companies do it is surely to establish a competitive advantage. In other words, they produce cost-effectiveness evaluations to show that their product has some unique value that the price paid ought to reflect. On the other side of the fence, the monopoly purchasers, particularly in Europe, are more interested in using the same evidence as a means of establishing a rather narrow purchasing platform – a 'best buy'. Therefore, there is a different motivation that makes it very hard to answer the question as put.

References

Danzon P and Furukawa M (2003) Prices and availability of pharmaceuticals: evidence from nine countries. *Health Affairs* Web Exclusive, October. Available from:
www.healthaffairs.org/WebExclusives/Danzon_Web_Excl_102903.htm (accessed 29 October 2003).
Danzon P, Wang R and Wang L (2005) The impact of price regulation on the launch delay of new drugs. *Health Economics* **14**: 269–92.

Index

ABPI *see* Association of the British Pharmaceutical Industry

AEP (Average European Price) system 65–6

age related macular degeneration (ARMD) 4

Agency for Medical Technology Assessment (ANAES) 8

Agenzia Italiana del Farmaco (AIFA) 64, 65, 66, 72, 73, 76

All-Wales Medicines Strategy Group (AWMSG) 42

ambulatory care 22, 23

ANAES *see* Agency for Medical Technology Assessment

Anatomical Therapeutic Chemical Classification System (ATC) 35

Andalusia, Spain xvi, 80, 83, 87

antibiotics 12

ARMD (age related macular degeneration) 4

Article 100 (Spain) 93–4

ASMR *see* Improvement in the Rendered Medical Service

Association of the British Pharmaceutical Industry (ABPI) 42, 44

ATC (Anatomical Therapeutic Chemical Classification System) 35

Australia 104

Austria 40, 41, 45

Average European Price (AEP) system 65–6

AWMSG *see* All-Wales Medicines Strategy Group

Basque Country, Spain 83

Belgium 40, 41, 45, 103, 104

benchmarking 52, 105

bio-equivalence of generics 107–8

biologics xv

Bismarckian schemes 21

Bouvenot, Professor Gilles 8

branded generics 74, 97, 98, 107

branded medicines
    bio-equivalence of generics 108
    international price comparisons 97, 98, 99
    Italy 74
    pricing for on-patent brands 105–6
    savings in generic market 106, 107
    Spain 88
    UK 40, 41, 42–3, 55

budgets
    Germany 23, 25, 30, 36–7
    Italy 63, 66, 73